SCOPE® MANUAL ON NUTRITION

MICHAEL C. LATHAM, M.D.
ROBERT B. McGANDY, M.D.
MARY B. McCANN, M.D.
FREDRICK J. STARE, M.D.

The Department of Nutrition
School of Public Health
Harvard University

PUBLISHED BY THE UPJOHN COMPANY, KALAMAZOO, MICHIGAN

Baird A. Thomas
Editor

Table of Contents

Preface

Fredrick J. Stare, M.D.
Professor of Nutrition
Chairman, Department of Nutrition

Our major job has been, and is, teaching, training, researching, and sending "our products" elsewhere to teach, train, research, and be of service in nutrition, which we consider an important and a largely neglected field of health and medicine. When the idea, and then the first draft of this Manual of Nutrition was born, my three collaborators were all young physician-nutritionists, members of Harvard's Department of Nutrition. But before this Manual was completed, two of my associates had left us. Dr. Michael Latham is now Professor of International Nutrition at Cornell University in Ithaca, New York and Dr. Mary B. McCann after a brief period with the United States Public Health Service in a position of key responsibility relative to the nutrition surveys conducted in ten states is now Professor of Nutrition and Chairman of the department at Teachers College, Columbia University. I am indebted to both of them for their help, particularly Dr. Latham who has continued to do more than his share.

Dr. Robert B. McGandy was an Associate Professor of Nutrition with us and played an important role in the preparation of the final draft for the first printing of this Manual. But he also has now left our department and is an Associate Professor of Physiology at the Harvard School of Public Health and a resident in pathology at the Boston City Hospital. Other members of Harvard's Department of Nutrition – Drs. D. S. Bernstein, Bernard Lown, Robert P. Geyer, George R. Kerr, K. C. Hayes, Phin Cohen, M. G. Herrera, and Jelia Witschi have had a hand in either writing or reading various sections of this Manual.

We all hope that this Manual, which is not a textbook, not a reference book, but a manual on nutrition primarily for medical, dental and other health students, house officers, and practitioners of medicine and dentistry, will teach a little nutrition and stimulate considerable interest in learning more nutrition and its application to problems of contemporary medicine and health.

Introduction

Nutrition is an important factor in health and in the etiology and management of several of the major causes of death and disability in our contemporary society. Atherosclerotic vascular disease, obesity, tooth decay, osteoporosis, and diabetes are common diseases in which nutrition is closely involved.

In the developing areas of the world, malnutrition of early childhood due to protein-calorie deficiencies as well as a host of infectious diseases made worse by poor nutrition, iodine deficiency goiter and blindness due to lack of vitamin A are a few major health problems directly related to inadequate nutrition.

Iron deficiency anemia and dental caries are widespread problems of inadequate nutrition which have neither geographic nor socio-economic boundaries. Even in highly developed societies, there may be large segments of the population in which hunger and undernutrition impair physical and mental performance.

As yet, instruction in the principles and practice of proper nutrition remains almost nonexistent in most of our medical, dental, public health and nursing schools today. The biochemical and physiological basis of nutrition is frequently no longer a part of the pre-clinical sciences. Clinically the major emphasis has been placed more on drugs and surgery than on the nutritional aspects of management and almost no attention is paid to the role of nutrition in the prevention of illness, and the improvement of health.

What is nutrition?

Nutrition is the science of food, the materials or nutrients in food, what they do and how they interact–all in relation to health. Nutrition comes from food, good food that one enjoys (for eating has always been one of the pleasures of life); from food in variety so that it supplies all of the 50-some known nutrients that are necessary for proper nutrition so as to provide the best of health that one's genetic or hereditary background permits.

Variety in foods consumed is the keystone to proper nutrition because no single food provides all the known nutrients, not even mothers' milk. Consuming no more calories than required to reach and maintain a desirable body weight is also important. This depends in large part on one's physical activities because muscular activities are the only way one has of using up calories beyond those needed for basal metabolism, doing your job well and whatever you do with leisure or spare time.

In the last decade or so, as will be pointed out later in this manual, it has been found that the caloric balance, the type of fat in the diet, as well as the cholesterol content of the diet are important factors affecting the level of cholesterol in the blood. The latter is one of the factors, and a most important one, in affecting susceptibility to coronary heart disease and cerebral hemorrhage. The higher the level of cholesterol (and also other fats) in the blood, the greater the chances of developing these common causes of death, particularly when it is in association with other conditions such as an elevated blood pressure, family history of death before life expectancy, diabetes, cigarette smoking, overweight, lethargy or infrequent physical activity.

Nutrition as a science can be divided into six main categories—protein, carbohydrate, fat, minerals, vitamins and water. The first three categories are the only ones that provide calories; that is, protein, carbohy-drate and fat. Four calories per gram are provided by both protein and carbohydrate. Fat provides slightly more than twice as much, 9 calories per gram.

Alcohol is not considered a foodstuff but from time immemorial it has been consumed by man in various fermented and distilled beverages and it does supply about 7 calories per gram so it must be considered in evaluating one's total caloric intake.

Minerals and vitamins provide no calories but function in the many metabolic processes whereby one obtains and utilizes energy from foods, builds and then maintains body tissues. Minerals also function as vital constituents of many body tissues such as the iron of hemoglobin, myoglobin, the cytochromes and the calcium and fluoride of sound teeth and bones.

Water, in addition to making up some 70% of the total body, is essential for the absorption of many nutrients, the elimination of body wastes via the urine and feces, and the maintenance of a normal body temperature via evaporation of water from the lungs and skin. While water provides no calories or vitamins it may provide calcium and magnesium in the case of "hard" waters and when fluoridated, either naturally or artificially, is the only important source of the mineral nutrient fluoride. This mineral nutrient is not only the single most important factor in lessening tooth decay (by 60-70%) but is important in lessening the incidence of osteoporosis in ageing and it may be important in lessening the incidence and severity of soft tissue calcification as for example in hardening of the arteries.

Nutrition is important in modern health and medicine—in improving and maintaining good health and in improving poor health. It is hoped that this manual will stimulate students of the health professions—medicine, dental, public health and nursing—as well as practitioners of the health professions, to learn more about nutrition and apply it for the benefit of mankind.

How prevalent is malnutrition in the USA?

This depends in part on what we mean by malnutrition. If we mean illness or poor health resulting in part from poor nutrition, it is widespread and among all economic classes. For here we would include tooth decay due to inadequate intake of the mineral nutrient, fluoride, and tooth decay is almost universal. We would include osteoporosis contributed to by lack of fluoride and this is radiologically demonstrable in 50% of adults over sixty years of age.

Related in part to malnutrition is atherosclerosis as manifested by coronary heart disease, cerebral, renal and peripheral artery disease. Essential hypertension can be lessened by decreasing the intake of the mineral nutrient sodium, and may possibly be caused by too much sodium and aggravated by obesity. These cardiovascular diseases are responsible for well over half the deaths in this country. Iron deficiency anemia is certainly prevalent in all societies.

The acute and severe vitamin deficiencies as manifested by the classical nutritional diseases—scurvy, pellagra, beriberi and xerophthalmia—are not common in the USA, but they are prevalent in many parts of the world. Vitamin deficiencies however, are prevalent in a large number of alcoholics in our country.

We have few data as to whether mild deficiencies of these vitamins or other nutrients are prevalent in the USA and particularly if they are responsible for manifestations of ill health.

Extensive nutritional surveys in the USA to evaluate health in relation to nutrient intake have been completed in ten states.[1] It is important that techniques for such studies be improved, deal with more nutrients, and the studies extended to provide factual data on the extent of malnutrition, not only among underprivileged people but also among privileged, and especially among young children. There should be a continued monitoring of the nutritional status of representative groups of our people. Infant mortality rates in the USA are higher than in fifteen other nations and we do not know the contribution of malnutrition to these deaths, but we do know that the death rates are higher among minority groups whose diets tend to be poor.

That there is something wrong with our food distribution system is clear. In the same city it is quite common to find school meals provided in the affluent suburbs but not in the ghetto sections. Food stamps are sometimes available, but frequently the money to buy the stamps is not. Surplus food distribution has been designed much more to help the producer of surplus foods than the poverty stricken consumer.

We do not know how often an empty belly leads individual Americans into crime or what the contribution of anxiety is to violence and rioting among people having insufficient food. We do not yet know the role that malnutrition plays in mental and behavioral development of children.

We do know that all is not well nutritionally in this most affluent of nations. Improved nutrition allied with other measures of health and social justice can make America a better place for all her citizens. It can solve the problems of overnutrition—of too many cal-

1. Ten-State Nutrition Survey 1968-1970, DHEW Pub. No. (HSM) 72-8134, 1972. CDC, Atlanta, Ga. 30333.

ories, of too much saturated fat—in the affluent and of nutritional deficiencies and varying degrees of starvation in the poor, the alcoholics, the aged, the senile, and the dejected.

Interest in nutrition as an important environmental factor in the health of man is increasing and rapidly. This stems from many directions, such as the realization that tooth decay, one of our most prevalent diseases, can be reduced by half or more via the adjustment (usually upward) of the mineral nutrient fluoride in community waters, a process known as fluoridation; that lowering the cholesterol level of the blood lessens the chances of developing coronary heart disease or a stroke; that essential hypertension can frequently be treated simply by a modest loss of weight and a generous decrease in the intake of sodium; that iron deficiency anemia is prevalent in about one-fourth of our total population. It is a noted fact that obesity is widely prevalent in our country and that while by itself and when only moderate it may not be a health hazard, yet it seldom exists by itself and then it is a real hazard to health; and finally the knowledge that undernutrition as a partner of poverty is far more prevalent than had been expected.

But here too progress has been made in recent years (and months) stemming largely from the White House Conference on Food and Nutrition. This conference was held in Washington, D.C., in early December, 1969, and incidentally, was organized and chaired by a member of Harvard's Department of Nutrition, Professor Jean Mayer. Among the conference recommendations that have in varying degrees been carried out are the following:

Liberalization of the Food Stamp Program: the amount allowable per family has been increased. The cost of stamps has been decreased (down to nothing for families with no resources). The coverage has gone up from about 2 million persons in 1969 to 13 million in 1972.

Improvement of the Commodities program: the number of commodities given every month used to number often no more than 5 or 6; the average is now 18, which permits a more balanced diet.

Meals-on-Wheels and Community Meals for the Elderly: a federal program now finances state, local, and private programs in both of these areas.

Enlargement of the School Lunch Program: about 8.5 million poor children now receive free school lunches (as compared to 4 million in 1969). Several hundred thousand free school breakfasts are also served daily.

Supplementary feeding program for pregnant and nursing women.

Consumer programs: a variety of measures have been undertaken or are being extensively tested. These include open dating of perishable commodities, unit pricing, nutritional labelling and a review of procedures on the safety of additives.

Education programs: a number of education measures ranging from nutrition education programs conducted by various food industries to the introduction of bills to support a Chair of Nutrition in every U.S. medical school.

This manual is not a textbook of nutrition. Several areas of medicine where nutrition is of importance such as diabetes, have been omitted because there already are excellent manuals on the nutritional aspects of these subjects or good chapters in standard medical texts. This is simply a manual on nutrition designed to interest the medical student and others interested in nutrition about the health of man today.

Fatty infiltration of the liver in kwashiorkor.
Michael C. Latham, M.D.

Recommended Dietary Allowances of Nutrients

This manual has been prepared primarily for use by medical students and physicians in the United States. Following is part of the introduction to the publication, Recommended Dietary Allowances,[1a] which is a report of the Food and Nutrition Board, National Academy of Sciences — National Research Council of the United States. This publication provides the recommended daily dietary allowances of nutrients and gives an explanation of how these allowances are estimated.

"Since 1940, the Food and Nutrition Board has developed formulations of daily nutrient intakes which were judged to be adequate for the maintenance of good nutrition in the population of the United States. These formulations were designated 'Recommended Dietary Allowances' in order to indicate that they were value-judgments based on the existing knowledge of nutritional science and subject to revision as new knowledge became available. The allowances are intended to serve as goals toward which to aim in planning food supplies and as guides for the interpretation of food consumption records of groups of people. Actual nutritional status of groups of people or individuals must be judged on the basis of physical, biochemical, and clinical observations combined with observations on food or nutrient intakes. If the recommended allowances are used as reference standards for interpreting records of food consumption, it should not be assumed that food practices are necessarily poor or that malnutrition exists because the recommendations are not completely met.

"The first edition of Recommended Dietary Allowances was published in 1943. The allowances recommended are those which, in the opinion of the Food and Nutrition Board, will maintain good nutrition in essentially all healthy persons in the United States under current conditions of living.

"The physiological and biochemical bases for the recommended allowances of each specific nutrient are described in the text. For proper understanding, application, and interpretation of the recommended allowances, it is necessary to appreciate how the allowances are related to estimates of average physiological requirements.

"The allowances are designed to afford a margin of sufficiency above average physiological requirements to cover variations among essentially all individuals in the general population. They provide a buffer against the increased needs during common stresses and permit full realization of growth and productive potential; but they are not to be considered adequate to meet additional requirements of persons depleted by disease or traumatic stresses. On the other hand, the allowances are generous with respect to temporary emergency feeding of large groups under conditions of limited food supply and physical disaster.

1a. *Recommended Dietary Allowances,* 7th Edition, NAS-NRC, Publication 1694, Washington, D.C., 1968. It is anticipated that the 8th Edition of this very useful publication will appear late in 1973 and that any changes from the 7th Edition will be minor.

"The margin of sufficiency above normal physiological requirements is different for each nutrient because of differences in the body storage capacity, in the range of individual requirements, in the precision of assessing requirements, and in the possible hazard of excessive intake of certain nutrients.

"Patterns of food consumption and food supplies in the United States permit ready adaptation to and compliance with the recommended allowances. The final objective of the recommended allowances is to permit and to encourage the development of food practices by the population of the United States that will allow for greatest dividends in health and in disease prevention."

The recommended dietary allowances therefore provide guidelines for the evaluation and development of diets for people in the United States. It should be clearly understood that the values presented are not requirements since many individuals are known to consume smaller amounts than those listed and still enjoy good health. On the other hand it is recognized that the actual requirement is not precisely known for any nutrient and the experimental estimates of requirements always show rather large differences in different experiments and in different individuals. The cause of these variations is generally unknown. No doubt they are partially explained by technical differences or errors of measurement and partly by actual differences in requirements among individuals which may be of genetic origin. When the true requirement is unknown, there is safety in recommending levels of nutrient intake above the estimated minimal need. The recommended dietary allowances therefore must not be considered actual requirements but rather levels of intake which should be entirely adequate for essentially all members of the population. This kind of dietary guidance seems appropriate in an affluent country such as the United States. It may not be appropriate in many parts of the world where more urgent problems exist and where food and money are more limiting factors for many people.

The presentation of one figure as a recommended intake for a particular group as in table I is likely to be somewhat misleading and often misinterpreted. The publication from which it is taken[2] provides explanations and justifications for values presented. The text should be consulted by those who are using the table.

It should be pointed out that the Recommended Dietary Allowances in the various editions are not the same, and never have been, as the Minimum Daily Requirements set forth by the Food and Drug Administration. The latter were usual many years ago in an attempt to try and actually maintain minimum daily requirements. They are now completely out of date, with no evidence to justify their continued use.

2. *Recommended Dietary Allowances*, 7th Edition, NAS-NRC, Publication 1694, Washington, D.C.,1968.

Special Medical Problems with a Nutritional Component

Nutritional Concepts in Heart Disease

I. THE USE OF NUTRITION IN THE PREVENTION OF ATHEROSCLEROTIC CARDIOVASCULAR DISEASE

Atherosclerotic vascular disease involving the coronary and cerebral circulation is the leading cause of death in the United States today. The disabilities among survivors of myocardial and cerebral infarction comprise problems of enormous magnitude to the socio-economic and medical aspects of individual care. Coronary heart disease is, in fact, becoming more frequent among men in the fourth and fifth decades of life. The magnitude of the problem of atherosclerosis, beginning in the second decade of life in over-nourished societies, and the premature mortality associated with coronary heart disease demand large scale preventive measures to reduce overall incidence and death rates.[3] Current medical practice cannot significantly mitigate morbidity and mortality from these causes.

Present concepts of atherosclerotic vascular disease suggest that a number of environmental influences interact with host factors in the progression and ultimate clinical manifestations. It is quite apparent that this disease is not the inevitable consequence of either age or of hereditary tendencies *per se*. Comprehensive evaluation of the evidence from clinical, pathological, epidemiological, and experimental animal studies suggests multifactorial causation. Diet, through its influence on lipid metabolism and circulating lipids, is an important environmental element. Other factors associated with coronary heart disease are hypertension, cigarette smoking, adiposity and

physical inactivity. The latter two are clearly interrelated. Resolution and understanding of the contributions and interactions of these factors as related to accelerated, premature clinical manifestations of atherosclerotic vascular disease have proved unhappily difficult. Even the extensive descriptive population studies cannot provide all the answers. Ultimate cellular and biochemical mechanisms are obscure. An adequate experimental animal model for the investigation of atherosclerosis and its clinical sequelae in man is not available.

Of all the basic regulating factors known to be associated with the disease which can be realistically manipulated to prevent or at least retard the atherosclerotic process, nutrition stands out. Elevation of blood lipids, particularly the induction of hyper beta-lipoproteinemia, is mandatory for the production of atherosclerosis in experimental animals. Dietary manipulation is the easiest way to achieve experimental atherogenesis. The extraordinary differences in blood lipids among peoples of various areas of the world are correlated with cardiovascular disease mortality. Differences in lipid distributions are related to dietary practices. The association of accelerated development of atherosclerosis and coronary heart disease with metabolic disorders in which circulating lipids are elevated has long been recognized. It has been a major contribution of the large, descriptive, epidemiologic study to demonstrate a quantitative association between lipids and the subsequent incidence of coronary and thrombotic cerebrovascular disease. The relationship shown in Chart 1a is typical of the association found in population studies.

To demonstrate relationships between factors and

---

3. Report of Inter-Society Commission for Heart Disease Resources. *Circulation* 42:53, 1970.

specific disease does not prove unique causality. The only proper way to identify causality in man is to carry out a controlled clinical trial designed to assess risk of disease in an appropriately sampled group in whom a factor associated with risk has been manipulated. A suitable study design, properly controlled is mandatory.

Of all the factors related to atherosclerotic vascular diseases aside from controlling hypertension, even mild hypertension, dietary changes to reduce blood lipids are more practical and effective than is intervention in other risk factors considering the lamentable status of our ability to motivate people to alter their life style. Persistent weight reduction, alteration of smoking habits, changing patterns of physical activity are very difficult to achieve in most individuals. Today there is increasingly secure evidence from clinical trials that dietary changes aimed at reducing the levels of serum lipids, especially cholesterol, can significantly reduce the incidence of coronary heart disease in man. One such study, a longitudinal evaluation of approximately 1,000 high risk individuals whose average serum cholesterol was reduced by 12% through diet alone has shown a significant reduction in coronary heart disease compared to a matched control group.[3a] Another controlled trial,[4] using men who had survived a myocardial infarction, has shown that the group treated with a lipid controlled diet had a significantly reduced incidence of myocardial re-infarction and angina pectoris over a five-year follow-up period compared to the counterpart control group. The average reduction in serum cholesterol in the diet-controlled groups was 17%.

3a. Christakis, G. et al., Am. J. Pub. Health 56:299, 1966.
 4. Leren, P., Circulation 42:935, 1970.

Chart 1a

Relative Risks of Developing Coronary Heart Disease According to Initial Serum Cholesterol Levels *men initially aged 30-59 years and followed up for 10 years.*

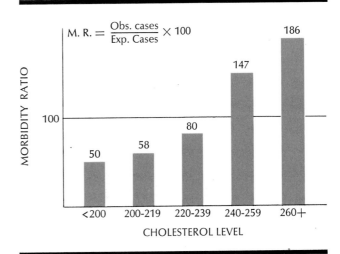

$$M.R. = \frac{Obs.\ cases}{Exp.\ Cases} \times 100$$

Chart 1b

NUMBER ONE KILLER — 1968

1. Analysis of Causes of Deaths

   a. Arteriosclerosis deaths
      Ischemic heart disease 677,260
      Chronic disease of endocardium &
      other myocardial insufficiency 7,630
      Cerebrovascular disease 209,420
      Arteriosclerosis 33,350
                   927,660

   b. Hypertension deaths
      Hypertension heart disease 10,000
      Hypertensive heart & renal disease 7,600
      Hypertension 8,980
                   26,580

     Total arteriosclerosis and
     hypertension deaths 954,240

   c. Deaths from other cardiovascular diseases
      Acute rheumatic fever & chronic
      rheumatic heart disease 16,440
      All other forms of heart disease .. 26,430
      Other diseases of arteries,
      arterioles and capillaries 24,270
                   67,140

   Total estimated deaths,
   cardiovascular diseases, 1968 1,021,380
   Total estimated deaths,
   all causes, 1968 1,923,000

2. 49.6% of All Deaths in 1968 Were Caused by Arteriosclerosis and Hypertension. Cardiovascular Diseases, as a Whole, Accounted for Over 53% of all Deaths.

Adapted from compilation of the National Health Education Committee, Inc., New York, N. Y. 10017

17

The aims of dietary management for the reduction of serum cholesterol are fourfold:

1. Adjust the calorie balance[5] to insure a desirable weight; modest restriction of caloric intake and modest increases in the level of physical activity will achieve this.

2. Lower the intake of saturated fat. The principal sources of saturated fat in the usual diet are from meats and dairy products. A lowered intake can be achieved by the careful selection, trimming of fat and portion size of meats and by emphasizing the increased use of fish and poultry which are naturally low in their content of saturated fat. Low fat dairy products—skimmed milk, low fat milks, cottage cheeses, sherbets—can be substituted for their high fat counterparts. The use of high fat baked products, including snacks, should be lessened unless the fat is a polyunsaturated fat.

3. Lower the intake of dietary cholesterol. The usual dietary intake of 600 to 800 mg. per day can be cut in half by limiting the use of egg yolks to two or three per week. Lessening the consumption of organ meats such as liver and shell fish and increasing the use of leaner meats and lower fat dairy products will also help to limit the cholesterol intake.

4. Raise the intake of polyunsaturated fats. These are found in abundance in corn, soya, safflower and cottonseed oils. Margarines, salad, cooking oils and shortenings made with these oils offer a substitute for animal fats which will maintain the daily fat intake at palatably high levels and contribute to a reduction in serum cholesterol.

Following these guidelines will lead to a modest reduction in the overall level of daily fat calories, from the 40 to 45% in usual diets to a level of 35 to 40%; the ratio of polyunsaturated to saturated fat will be raised to 1:1 or higher.

NOTE ON CIRCULATING LIPIDS

The beta lipoproteins (complexes of triglyceride, cholesterol, and phospholipid wrapped in carrier protein) are the agents most closely associated with atherosclerosis–both in laboratory animals and in man. The measurements of total plasma cholesterol and of fasting triglyceride provide useful though indirect estimates of the level of the beta lipoproteins. While knowledge of cholesterol and triglyceride alone is sufficient for screening and for assessing management in the great proportion of the population, among the 5 per cent of middle-aged individuals with a plasma cholesterol of 300 mg. per 100 ml. or above or with a lactescent fasting serum, determination of electrophoretic or physical-chemical properties of the lipoproteins[6] is important to their management.

5. The American Heart Association, 44 East 23rd Street, New York, New York 10010 has available additional information on modified fat diets.
6. Fredrickson, D. S., Levy, R. I., and Lees, R. S., New Eng. J. Med. 276:34, 94, 148, 215, 273, 1967.

II. NUTRITIONAL THERAPY OF CONGESTIVE HEART FAILURE AND HYPERTENSION

Reduction of body sodium by dietary restriction and pharmacologic intervention are the aims of current nutritional therapy of heart failure and hypertension. Net body loss of sodium in the individual with a failing heart reduces extracellular fluid volume, correcting edema and its complications, and reducing circulating fluid volume, all lessening the work of the heart. The resulting improvement of organ perfusion, especially of the kidneys, results in the ability of intrinsic homeostatic mechanisms to regain control of sodium balance, and improves exercise tolerance.

Today's physician is becoming increasingly aware that the natriuretic drugs, the diuretics and cardiac glycosides, are not without hazard, and, lamentably, not infrequently have had fatal consequences. Effective diuretics are associated with potassium as well as sodium loss. Potassium depletion secondary to diuretic therapy increases myocardial irritability and predisposes to threatening arrhythmias. This compromise is potentiated by the cardiac glycosides, drugs used frequently in combination with the potassium-depleting diuretics. Too frequently drugs are employed in the treatment of patients who would respond to dietary sodium restriction alone, if prescribed with the same conviction.

The aim of nutritional therapy is to induce negative sodium balance in the body. The physician prescribes a diet which is adequate nutritionally but restricted in its sodium content. Usual sodium ion intake for an American has been estimated at 3-7 gm. or 150-300 mEq. per day. Therapeutic regimens range from the "no added salt diet," approximately 2.3 gm. sodium (100 mEq./Na.), to as low as 230 mg. sodium (10 mEq.) per day.

Patients frequently misunderstand the sources of salt or sodium in the diet. It should be the responsibility of the physician to insure that the patient understands that foods *naturally* contain sodium. The most understandable explanation is that just as we retain sodium in our bodies, so does the animal, and therefore foods of animal origin–meat, milk, cheese and butter— are major sources of dietary sodium. The processes of preservation of foods often necessitate the addition of salt, and thus many smoked, cured and canned foods contain high concentrations of sodium. Many food condiments and flavor enhancers contain sodium in the form of monosodium glutamate (MSG). Food tables are available which provide information on the amount of sodium contained in common foods, expressed usually in milligrams [with 1 mEq. equal to 23 mg.Na.(Appendix A)]. (The American Heart Association can provide the physician with excellent materials for patient distribution.)

It is true that diuretics and cardiac glycosides are among our most potent therapeutic tools in dealing with a patient with heart failure, and are definitely indicated in addition to dietary sodium restriction in the severely compromised patient. If there exists a clinical necessity for the use of these drugs together, or of the diuretics alone, potassium supplementation must be instituted. Potassium salts are gastric irritants and are unpalatable, causing nausea, vomiting, and rejection by the patient. This is why potassium salts have been given as enteric coated tablets. This preparation may cause ulceration of the small intestine and its unhappy consequences. If potassium supplementation is necessary, potassium-rich foods are an economical, palatable, and a simple approach contrasted with potassium elixers. Especially with these preparations the possibility of overdosage must be considered, another probable fatal result of the failure to recognize the safer nutritional approach.

Patients on diuretic therapy may require potassium ion intakes as high as 5 gm. (130 mEq.) per day. A list of foods which contain concentrated amounts of potassium is found in Appendix A. The nutritional approach to sodium restriction and potassium supplementation cannot be understated as important adjuncts for the patient requiring manipulation of electrolyte balance.

Obesity

A type of malnutrition which is highly prevalent and readily visible, is obesity, often the by-product of affluence and of a way of life in which the levels of caloric intake and energy expenditure are unbalanced. Aside from the often serious social and psychological stigma created by obesity, it is also associated with an increased risk of many diseases and of aggravating others; gross obesity generally shortens the life span itself. Cardiovascular and pulmonary diseases, hypertension, diabetes, cholelithiasis, peripheral vascular and orthopedic disorders are among the medical hazards linked to or aggravated by adiposity. Within the present capacity of the physician, the treatment of obesity is often discouraging. It is the nature of obesity to perpetuate itself. Thus, it may well be that *prevention* of excessive weight gain will offer the most effective and practical approach to the problem.

Figure 1
Triceps skinfold thickness measured by a skinfold caliper. Duplicate measurements should be obtained for an average measurement of adipose tissue.

Definitions and Assessment

The terms obesity and overweight are not synonymous; the former denotes an excess of adipose tissue; the latter makes no distinction among the several body components, muscle, bone, or fat. Body fluid is not considered. An individual may be overweight relative to some arbitrary standard and yet not be obese. While football players are the classically cited examples of this, such instances are not often found among the general, middle-aged population. By measuring weight for height and comparing this to standards approximate to sex and age, one is not necessarily able to qualify an individual on the continuum of adiposity. Gross overweight usually implies gross obesity; such individuals clearly have a risk of increased morbidity and mortality from major diseases. But the relative risks of lesser degrees of overweight are not clear and it is probably the measurement of adiposity that is relevant in this regard.

Total adipose tissue cannot be conveniently or directly measured, but the determination of skinfold thickness at standard sites does offer a simple method for quantitating adiposity. Such estimates are highly correlated with total body fat; constant pressure skinfold calipers allow the physician to make these measurements reliably. The triceps and subscapular skinfolds are the sites generally used. The former is more easily obtained and gives more reproducible results. With the right arm flexed at 90°, a tape measure is used to accurately locate on the back of the triceps the midpoint between tip of the acromion and olecranon. The caliper is applied to the fold of skin pulled away at this location. Upper limits of normal values for a healthy Caucasian American population are shown in Appendix D.

Height-weight tables have been the most commonly used standards for quantitating overnutrition; their limitations have already been mentioned. The tables of desirable or ideal weight (for sex and weight) represent those weights of insurees with optimal mortality experience (Appendix D). For many obese middle-aged patients, these weights represent goals which are discouragingly beyond achieving.

Height, weight, skinfold thickness, an appraisal of an individual's general appearance, an evaluation of his own motivation and goals provide the basis for a meaningful evaluation of obesity and for a realistic attempt at a successful treatment.

Among women, increases in adipose tissue are most marked during pregnancies and after the menopause. Males tend to acquire adipose tissue at a more constant rate from the third decade onward. Obese children and adolescents are a major reservoir for relatively intractable obesity in adult life; they usually have much more difficulty in achieving and maintaining weight reduction as adults.

Treatment and Prevention

The difficulties encountered with treatment strongly suggest a concern for the *prevention* of obesity. The major focus on preventive measures ought to be in adolescence and early adulthood. The long term aim of either treatment or prevention is to instill a sensible program of dietary *and exercise* habits which will assure stable energy balance throughout life.

Diet

A proper therapeutic diet for obesity should provide all necessary nutrients in sufficient amounts and be restricted in caloric content. It should be palatable and easily available from the viewpoint of economics and convenience. The patient should be educated so that once desired weight has been achieved, minor changes, such as increasing portion size of foods allowed, will provide a proper maintenance diet. The caloric deficit desired can be estimated from the fact that a pound of body fat respresents the equivalent of about 3500 calories. Thus a daily deficit of 500 calories will lead to an average weekly loss of one pound. In relatively active patients, a daily intake of less than 1500 calories for men and 1000 for women is poorly tolerated. Increased physical activity can help in-

crease the caloric deficit so that a patient can obtain a total deficit of 500 calories per day without cutting food intake to this extent. Thus a decrease in calories from food and drink of 300 per day and an increase in caloric expenditure of 200 calories per day will accomplish the same effect as a decrease of 500 calories in the diet and be more acceptable to most people.

Experience has shown that a balanced diet with 12-14 per cent of calories as protein, 35 to 40 per cent in fat calories, a reduction in saturated fats, with the remaining calories supplied by carbohydrate, all provided by foods of sufficient variety, is the best diet over a long period of time. There is no evidence that more extreme diets, especially fad diets, which constantly appear and/or disappear have any advantage over a calorically restricted, balanced, "normal" diet. Moreover fad diets do not provide realistic programs which can be followed for the necessary period of time needed to maintain body weight, and some of them are actually dangerous to health.

The chief advantage of "formula diets" which became popular during the past decade is that they provide a simple, rigid regimen that does not need to be based on any knowledge of food and food values. They may be useful at the beginning of a weight control program or for a one-meal a day replacement in certain instances.

Bulk-producing agents such as methyl cellulose have not been shown to be of any special merit. Salads, fruits and vegetables are superior bulk-producing agents as well as being more palatable and more likely to become part of a lifelong dietary pattern.

Salt restriction is useful in obese subjects with a tendency to excessive fluid retention, particularly middle-aged and older women and sedentary persons. Salt restriction is a more sound measure than the use of diuretics to prevent excessive water retention.

Most appetite-depressant drugs are sympathomimetic amines related in structure to amphetamine. They act chiefly by stimulating the ventromedial (satiety) hypothalamic center, but may have other accessory actions, including stimulation of spontaneous physical activity and of free fatty acid release by adipose tissue. In most cases, the effective duration of amphetamine treatment is of the order of a month to six weeks. They are useful to tide a patient over periods of excessive hunger that persist in spite of meal and snack adjustment. Anorexigenic agents are most useful at the onset of treatment and with patients who have recently become obese.

Dessicated thyroid has been used as an adjunct to weight reduction on the grounds that obese patients are in a hypometabolic state and, therefore, can lose weight easier if metabolic stimulation is accomplished. Most obese patients, however, are euthyroid. Thyroid hormones in small doses suppress endogenous hormone production, resulting in no net effect. Larger doses produce a hyperthyroid state with its serious side effects, and cause loss of lean body mass rather than fat. The drug is not recommended for general use in weight reduction programs.

Repeated cycles of weight changes are an all too frequent result of crash programs and fad diets. Such cycles may be more harmful than the maintenance of a steady weight, even at levels of moderate obesity.

Exercise is a most important factor in a realistic reducing program. For most individuals, exercise is the great variable in energy expenditure, and reduction or elimination of exercise is not generally followed by a reduction in food intake. Conversely, exercise does not increase voluntary food intake in inactive subjects until it has reached a certain critical duration and intensity.

In general, the long-term results of a variety of weight reduction programs utilizing both individual and group approaches to weight control have been unhappily discouraging. Characteristically, once desired weight was achieved, therapy ceased, and weight was regained. Because maintenance of the new desirable weight requires a new pattern of eating and activity for the individual, it is highly probable that intermittent support following weight loss might prevent the common return to pre-dieting weight levels.

For further reading on the subject of obesity consult: U.S. Department of Health, Education and Welfare, U.S. Public Health Service's booklet on, "Obesity and Health," available from U.S. Government Printing Office, Washington, D.C. 20402.

Dental Caries

Dental caries is the most widespread disease in the United States. In some parts of the country as many as 90 percent of the population surveyed have serious dental problems requiring either tooth extractions or restorations. A complete loss of teeth early in adolescence is occasionally seen and by middle age is fairly common. Edentulous persons often have difficulty in consuming certain foods and this sometimes makes it hard for them to get a balanced diet. The dental profession does not have the trained manpower to provide adequate dental care to everyone. If poverty and lack of knowledge were not important factors in limiting the numbers seeking dental treatment then dentists would be overwhelmed and quite unable to cope with the dental pathology that would be presented to them. The prevention of dental caries by whatever means possible is therefore of great public health importance.

That modern western diets have had an effect on the prevalence of dental caries is shown by the much higher number of teeth that are decayed, missing and filled in groups of persons of the same age that are surveyed in the U.S. and many developing countries.

Figure 2a
Girl, age 15, drank water with very low fluoride content throughout life. Of 26 erupted secondary teeth, decayed (D)–2, missing (M)–2, and filled (F)–15 for DMF score of 19.

Figure 2b
Girl, age 15, from an adjoining community, drank water fluoridated to 1 ppm throughout life. Of 28 erupted secondary teeth, (D)–0, (M)–0, and (F)–6, for DMF score of 6, a reduction 68%.

It is almost certain that sticky adherent carbohydrate foods with a low rate of clearance from the oral cavity are an important factor in this respect.[7]

Many nutrients are necessary for the development of the teeth and surrounding structures. Vitamin A is important for normal bone growth. Inadequate growth patterns which result in orthodontic problems can result from vitamin A deficiency. The effects of a deficiency of vitamin C on the soft supporting tissues of the teeth have been described in the section dealing with scurvy. It should be noted that these gum lesions do not occur in the edentulous. Protein is also essential for the normal development of the teeth and supporting tissues.

Vitamin D, calcium and phosphorus which are important in bone development are also essential to the growth of the teeth. There is some controversy as to whether vitamin D supplementation helps to reduce caries-susceptibility. The general balance of evidence suggests that where inadequate quantities of vitamin

7. Shaw, J. H., in *Modern Nutrition in Health and Disease,* edited by Wohl and Goodhart, Lea and Febiger, Philadelphia, 1968.

D are obtained either from the diet or from exposure of the body to sunlight, then vitamin D taken orally will help reduce the caries rate.

However fluoride is the single most important mineral in relation to dental caries. In the 1930's it was observed that individuals who had access to drinking water that contained 1 to 2 parts per million (ppm) of fluoride had considerably less tooth decay than persons whose water supply had much lower amounts of fluoride. It was subsequently found that in areas where the water had very little fluoride it was possible to reduce the incidence of dental caries by 60 to 70 per cent by adjusting the fluoride level of the water to about 1 ppm. In 1945 a careful experimental trial was begun using three communities (Newburgh, New York; Brantford, Ontario; and Grand Rapids, Michigan) in which fluoride was added to the water. Three neighboring control cities were chosen with no fluoridation and where the fluoride content of the water was low. After ten years it was found that children who had been receiving fluoridated water from an early age had 60 to 70 per cent less dental caries

Chart 2

Reduction in Decayed, Missing and Filled Permanent Teeth) *(6 and 7 year-olds, 7 years after fluoridation)*

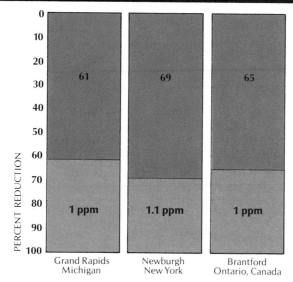

Dental examinations on 6 and 7 year-old children, seven years after the institution of fluoridation, have revealed a reduction of 61%, 69% and 65% in decayed, missing or filled teeth in Grand Rapids, Michigan; Newburgh, New York, and Brantford, Ontario, Canada, respectively.

Chart 4

Interaction of fluoride with the hydroxyapatite mineral lattice of the teeth.

$$3 \cdot Ca_3 P_2 O_8 \cdot Ca\ (OH)_2 \quad \text{HYDROXYAPATITE}$$
$$+2\ F^- \quad \text{(caries-susceptible)}$$
$$\downarrow$$
$$3\ Ca_3 P_2 O_8 \cdot Ca\ (F)_2 \quad \text{FLUORAPATITE}$$
$$+2\ OH^- \quad \text{(promotes caries-resistance)}$$

Chart 3

Decayed, Missing, and Filled Teeth* per Child
Ten Years After Fluoridation   *Permanent teeth

GRAND RAPIDS, MICHIGAN 1944
before fluoridation
GRAND RAPIDS, MICHIGAN 1954
10 years after fluoridation (1 ppm)
AURORA, ILLINOIS 1945
naturally fluoridated water (1.2 ppm)

This chart shows a reduction in dental caries of permanent teeth by 60-70 percent in children who consumed fluoridated water from birth versus those who were denied this important mineral nutrient.

than did the children in the other communities.[8] Trials in other cities and in several countries have given similar results. Today there are over 8600 communities serving over 95 million people that have fluoridated water in the United States.

There is no doubt that the fluoridation of water supplies is a public health measure of very great importance. It is the responsibility of every physician, dentist, and health worker to urge and support fluoridation of the water supply where needed. Generally the opponents of fluoridation fall into three categories. They are health faddists, those who for quasi-religious reasons are opposed to any type of medication, and those who equate fluoridation with an interference in their individual rights. Fluoridation has been found to be absolutely safe at one part per million (ppm) for people of all ages and in every state of health. Fluoridation is not a form of medication for it is an adjustment of the level of a nutrient just as is the fortification of bread with vitamins. Fluoridation is no more an infringement of freedom of individual rights than is the chlorination of water or the regulation of the speed limit.

There are substitutes for fluoridation such as pills, drops or fluoridated toothpaste but none combine the efficiency, the effectiveness and economy of fluoridation for the general public. The addition of fluoride to infant vitamin preparations is very useful because fluoride has its maximum effectiveness when received early in life. Especially when the infant is breast-fed, fluoride vitamin supplements are desirable, even in fluoride communities, because fluoride does not readily cross the mammary gland in adequate amounts. Such preparations are not contraindicated when fluoridated water is consumed but actually give added protection from dental decay.

8. Shaw, J. H., in *Modern Nutrition in Health and Disease,* edited by Wohl and Goodhart, Lea and Febiger, Philadelphia, 1968.

Chart 5

Incidence of Decayed and Filled Deciduous Teeth
(Three years after first dental examination)
Patient age approximately 7

	Number of Patients	% of Children with All Good Teeth	Mean No. of New Decayed & Filled Teeth
Infant Group (Fluoride-Vitamin from Birth)	108	60.2	0.98
Water Group (Fluoride in Water from Birth)	41	43.9	1.59
Baseline Group (Fluoride-Vitamin since Age 4)	277	30.3	2.14
Control Group (No Fluoride)	212	24.5	2.92

Infants started on fluoride from birth compared to a control group showed more than twice as many children with all good teeth at age seven. These same groups showed approximately one filled tooth in the fluoride group for every three in the child who had no fluoride.

There is a statistical difference (P < .01) between the "Control" and "Infant" group and between the "Infant" and "Baseline" group (P < .01) with the "Infant" group having a statistically higher percentage of children with all good teeth.   P = probability.

Chart 6

Decayed, Missing and Filled Teeth *of children 6-10 years old in fluoridated and non-fluoridated cities*

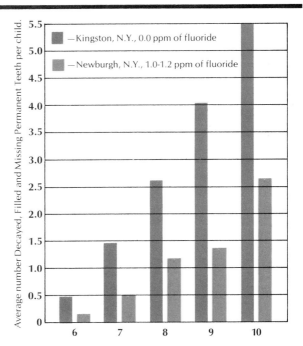

— Kingston, N.Y., 0.0 ppm of fluoride

— Newburgh, N.Y., 1.0-1.2 ppm of fluoride

Results from fluoridation in 6-10 year old children in Kingston, N. Y. (no fluoride) and Newburgh, N. Y. (1.0-1.2 ppm of fluoride).

Osteoporosis

Osteoporosis is a chronic disease of aging. It is extremely prevalent in the United States and as the population tends to live longer it is becoming ever more important.

The disease is characterized by an excessive demineralization of bone which is often responsible for considerable pain. This is commonly in the back and may radiate around the trunk and extend into the legs. It sometimes incapacitates the individual because the pain is aggravated by movement and by jarring the spine in walking. A frequent complication in the elderly is the fracturing of bones. This may be the collapse of one or more vertebrae, it may be the fracture of the hip due to a minor fall, or it may involve some other bone.

Osteoporosis is usually diagnosed radiologically. A good radiograph of the spine may be helpful but for survey purposes x-rays of the hand, wrist or jaw are more useful. There is in these areas less variability due to soft tissue and gas overlay of the bone. In all cases the shadow of the bone shows diminished density.

Full descriptions of osteoporosis appear in the standard medical textbooks. From a nutritional point of view there is new interest in the disease because evidence now indicates that fluoride is effective in the treatment of the disease[9] and may be important also in its prevention. It is known that fluoride becomes a part of the bone substance just as it does in dental enamel, replacing hydroxyl ions in the chemical composition of the bone and giving rise to a larger bone crystal which may be less liable to resorption.

The first evidence that fluoride intake might be an important factor in osteoporosis came from a comparison of x-rays taken in two communities, one of which had water with a low fluoride content and one with a high fluoride content. It was found that in the former community there was substantially more osteoporosis and decreased bone density.[10] A recent study was made in two comparable areas of North Dakota[11] which had differing amounts of fluoride in their water. Judged both by relative bone density and from the presence or absence of collapsed vertebrae there was substantially less osteoporosis in the high-fluoride areas.

Fluoride has now been used in the treatment of osteoporosis for a number of years with beneficial results. In treatment, doses have varied from 5 mg. to over 60 mg. of fluoride daily usually given as a sodium fluoride tablet. The daily dose necessary to produce remission is much larger than that which can be ingested from drinking fluoridated water. However, this does not mean that drinking fluoridated water from an early age may not help to substantially reduce osteoporosis in the elderly in the later years. This however remains to be proved.

There was a widely held belief that calcium deficiencies in the diets of the elderly were important in the causation of osteoporosis. This is now disputed[12] as there are no good studies to substantiate such a claim. Calcium has not been effective in the treatment of the disease and there is no sound epidemiological evidence to show that osteoporosis is more prevalent where deficient calcium diets are regularly eaten. In fact, osteoporosis has been shown to be an important problem in the United States, Great Britian and Scandinavia, three areas where calcium intakes tend to be rather high.

9. Bernstein, D. S. and Cohen, P., *J. Clin. Endocrinol. 27*:197, 1967.

10. Leone, N. C. *et al., Arch. Indust. Health 21*:326, 1960.
11. Bernstein, D. S., *et al., JAMA 198*:499, 1966.
12. Hegsted, D. M., *J. Am. Dietet. Assoc. 50*:105, 1967.

Iron Deficiency Anemia

Iron deficiency is one of the most common nutritional deficiencies in the United States. It occurs most frequently in infants beyond 6 months of age, in adolescent girls, and in women in the reproductive period. While good data on prevalence of iron deficiency in any group are not available, it is known to be high in some segments of the population. There are difficulties in defining iron deficiency. Presumably the sequence of events during iron depletion would be loss of iron stores (which may be estimated by staining marrow smears for iron), fall in plasma iron (normal = 50 μg./100 ml.), increase in iron-binding capacity of plasma (normally over 10% saturation), and, finally, development of anemia. In severe iron deficiency this is usually a hypochromic microcytic anemia. The frequency with which iron deficiency is encountered will depend upon the criteria used. Most often simple measurement of hemoglobin or hematocrit has been used. This will certainly underestimate the extent of iron depletion.

Iron is absorbed and excreted only with difficulty. In the usual adult male, 0.5 to 1.0 mg. of iron is lost daily. In the adult menstruating woman, the usual losses are twice as high, often even more, depending upon the amount of blood loss. Similarly, there appears to be great variation in the ability of individuals to absorb dietary iron. On the average, about 10% of the dietary iron is absorbed. An intake of 10 mg. of iron per day would be required to replace the loss of 1 mg. in the adult male and greater in the adult female. The situation is further complicated by the accumulating data showing that the availability of iron in foods may vary greatly. It has been reported that iron in wheat is poorly absorbed whereas that in meat is well absorbed. These differences might, however, be modified by the mixture of foods consumed.

A recent report indicated that egg yolk impairs the absorption of iron, this despite the fact that it is one of the better food sources of iron.[13]

In the adult, iron deficiency is frequently associated with blood loss. In many parts of the world excessive blood losses are associated with hookworm infestation, leading to serious iron deficiency anemia. High iron requirements are also associated with growth, iron being required for all cells and particularly for the increase in blood volume. Iron deficiency is frequently encountered in infancy, especially in infants born to anemic mothers. The normal infant is born with iron stores but milk is a very poor source of iron. Unless supplemented foods, rich in iron or supplements containing iron are provided, anemia will be common in the latter part of infancy and early childhood. Anemia and iron depletion may also be common in adolescent girls who bear the combined stress of growth and menstruation. Pregnancy also imposes the stress of the growth of the fetus combined with an expansion of the blood volume. With poor dietary habits, young girls and women may often enter pregnancy with reduced iron stores.

Variations in iron requirements and in iron utilization, make it difficult to estimate the iron requirement of any individual. The Recommended Dietary Allowances are set on the high side so that the needs of the majority will be met. The new allowances (1968) specify higher levels for women than previously and these levels will apparently not be met by the usual diets in the United States. The question is therefore posed, should the usual diet contain enough iron to meet the needs of individuals with high iron requirements? If so, how can this be accomplished? Most bread and flour in the United States is fortified with iron. The quantity should be increased. However,

13. Symposium: Iron Deficiency and Absorption, *Am. J. Clin. Nutr.* 21:1138, 1968.

women and girls do not ordinarily consume large amounts of bread. Thus foods other than bread should be considered for iron fortification.

Control of iron deficiency in the United States is complicated by the fact that total food intake becomes smaller as the population becomes more sedentary and many girls and women are concerned about obesity. When the total caloric intake is low and approximately 40% of the calories are supplied as fat and 15-20% as sugar, there is little room in the diet for iron-containing foods. Improved manufacturing methods, use of stainless and aluminum utensils and emphasis on cleanliness have lowered the total iron intake. Iron toxicity (hemosiderosis and hemochromatosis) exists, is rare, is probably hereditary, and is unlikely to be increased by more adequate fortification of foods with iron.

Protein-Calorie Malnutrition of Young Children

Protein-calorie malnutrition in young children constitutes the most important and widespread nutritional problem in the world today. The two main clinical syndromes are kwashiorkor and nutritional marasmus. In kwashiorkor the principal deficiency is of protein whereas in marasmus there is an overall deficit in food intake including calories and protein. From the clinical point of view there are many intermediate cases which are difficult to fit into either category and which have some of the symptoms and signs of both conditions.

It should be recalled that these clinical entities constitute only the relatively small exposed part of the enormous iceberg of protein-calorie malnutrition. There are perhaps 99 children who are receiving an inadequate diet, who are poorly grown and who are prone to infections for every frank case of serious clinical protein-calorie deficiency disease. These 99 children are mild or sub-clinical cases of protein-calorie malnutrition, and typically remain submerged in the population of children. They are liable to be precipitated into one of these clinical states by any of a variety of causes.

Over the past two decades kwashiorkor has been recognized and studied in many parts of the world. It is now accepted as one disease with a few local variations. During this period, the emphasis has been on protein deficiency and a world-wide effort has been made to increase the quantity and quality of protein available to children. More recently attention has turned to the equal importance of a shortage of calories as part of an overall deficiency of food in the diets of young children.

Kwashiorkor and nutritional marasmus can be regarded as the two extremes of protein-calorie malnutrition of young children. However, very many cases of protein-calorie malnutrition are intermediate and this has given rise to such names as "marasmic-kwashiorkor" in cases where kwashiorkor is superimposed on marasmus. A separate description is given kwashiorkor and of nutritional marasmus, but the clinician must expect many cases to be intermediate between the two extremes.

Figure 3a
Kwashiorkor—skin lesions.

KWASHIORKOR
Etiology and Epidemiology

Kwashiorkor occurs mainly in children 1 to 3 years of age. It is common in many developing countries of

Figure 3b
Kwashiorkor in an African child showing edema and dermatosis.

Asia, Africa and Latin America, but has been reported in Europe and the United States where it is associated with poverty.

The disease occurs in children whose diet is grossly deficient in protein. Often the food that the child is receiving is of a type which contains mainly carbohydrate and little protein. In many parts of the world it is a disease of the weaning period when the child is taken from the breast onto a mainly starchy diet. An adequate intake of breast milk will provide a satisfactory diet for the first four to six months of an infant's life. After that, mainly because of reduced quantities, breast milk provides merely a useful protein-rich dietary supplement to whatever other food the child is receiving.

Important factors often implicated in the complex etiology of kwashiorkor are:

(a) The rapid growth and relatively high protein requirements of the rapidly growing young child.

(b) A protein-poor, staple food for the child, e.g., manioc, bananas, sugar.

(c) Poor infant feeding practices.

(d) A lack of protein-rich foods both animal (meat, milk, fish, eggs, etc.) and vegetable (e.g., beans, peanuts, etc.).

(e) A poor distribution of available food in the family (e.g., the adults and older children often get the major share of protein-rich foods such as meat.).

(f) Seasonal food shortages.

(g) Poverty and its attendant ills.

(h) Cultural dietary practices including food taboos which may preclude the child consuming certain available and desirable foods.

(i) Infections such as diarrhea, measles, whooping cough, etc.

(j) Ignorance or lack of knowledge on the part of parents or guardians, on what foods are needed in the child's diet.

(k) Psychological factors which may affect the appetite of the child.

On The Way to Better Health

Figure 4a
Mealtime for hospitalized children in New Guinea.

Figure 4b
School lunch in a village in Tunisia.

Figure 4c
Supervised school lunch program in Thailand.

Figure 4d
School lunch in Massachusetts, U.S.A.

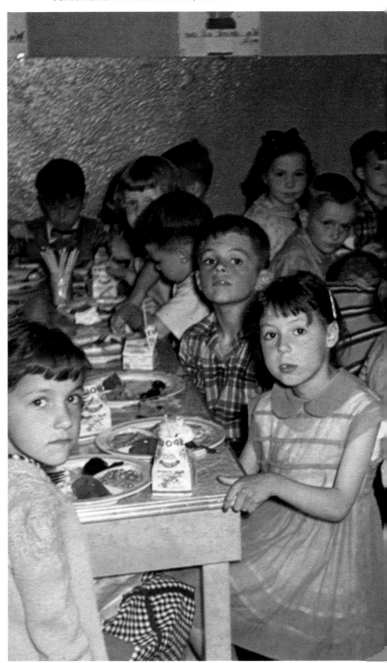

The Disease

The following are the main features of kwashiorkor:

(a) *Growth failure* which is always present. If the child's age is known he will be found to be shorter, and except in cases with gross edema, lighter than normal.

(b) *Wasting* is always a feature, but may be masked by edema. The wasting is often evident in the muscles of the arms and legs.

(c) *Edema* always occurs and is a most important feature of the disease. It may affect any part of the body. In an ambulant child it usually starts as a slight swelling of the feet which often spreads up the legs. Later the hands, scrotum and face may all be affected.

(d) *Mental changes* are invariably present. The child is usually apathetic and disinterested in his surroundings. At the same time he is miserable and irritable when being moved or disturbed. He is unsmiling and his behavioral development is retarded.

(e) *Hair changes*—In kwashiorkor the hair often shows changes in texture, in color, in strength, and in ease of pluckability. The tight curl of African or Afro-American hair is often lost, the hair becomes silkier and loses its lustre. Black hair becomes brown or reddish brown in color. In Latin America parallel strips of discolored hair have been labeled the "flag sign."

(f) *Skin changes*—These are not invariable, but if present may be very characteristic. The skin, especially of the face, may show depigmentation. In some cases a dermatosis develops especially in areas of friction such as the groins and behind the knees. Darkly pigmented patches appear and these may desquamate like old blistered paint, which has given rise to the term "flaky paint dermatosis." Beneath the flakes are atrophic areas which may resemble a healing burn.

(g) *Diarrhea*—Stools are frequently loose and contain undigested particles of food. Sometimes they are offensive, watery and blood-stained.

(h) *Anemia*—Most cases of kwashiorkor have some degree of anemia. This is due in part to a lack of protein to synthesize blood cells, but is frequently complicated by anemia due to iron deficiency, hookworm infestation, malaria, etc.

(i) *Hepatomegaly*—The liver may be palpably enlarged. This is due to fatty infiltration of the liver which is always found post mortem in kwashiorkor.

(j) *Signs of other deficiencies*—In kwashiorkor there is usually some sub-cutaneous fat present in contrast to marasmus where there is usually none or very little. The degree of its lack gives an indication of the degree of calorie deficiency. Lesions of the lips and mouth characteristic of vitamin B deficiencies may occur. Xerosis or xerophthalmia due to vitamin A deficiency may sometimes be present.

Laboratory findings

In kwashiorkor there is usually a reduction in total serum proteins with the serum albumin content reduced more than the globulin. Serum amylase and pancreatic enzymes are also reduced as well as the ratio of essential to non-essential amino acids. Serum transferrin levels are also low and the extent of the reduction gives a good index of the severity of the disease. Liver biopsy reveals fatty infiltration but despite the presence of edema there is no albumin in the urine.

Treatment

All severe cases should, if possible, be admitted to a hospital for treatment. Severity is judged by the amount of edema, the extent of dermatosis, the hemoglobin level, the severity of diarrhea, vomiting and dehydration, the willingness of the child to feed, but above all by the general clinical condition of the patient.

Dried skimmed milk is a most satisfactory basis for treatment, but other protein-rich foods are effective. A mixture of dried skimmed milk, vegatable oil and casein is ideal, and if necessary the child can be given the mixture through an intragastric tube. The milk mixture should provide about 120 calories and 7 gm. of protein per kilogram of body weight per day.

If diarrhea is severe, potassium should be administered at a dose of approximately 0.5 gm. potassium chloride in water three times a day.

Antibiotics should be given to combat infection. In malarial areas, chloroquine or some other antimalarial drug is also desirable.

When shock or severe anemia or dehydration occurs, appropriate supportive measures are indicated. In cases of shock or if the anemia is severe, a blood transfusion might prove life saving. Anemia of a moderate nature can be treated with oral or parenteral iron therapy.

Severe dehydration calls for the administration of intravenous electrolyte solutions.

Vitamins should be given for vitamin deficiences and it is especially important to treat any evidence of eye changes caused by vitamin A deficiency.

Severe cases of kwashiorkor can be expected to respond quite rapidly to the above regimen. The diarrhea and gastrointestinal symptoms subside, diuresis occurs with rapid reduction of edema and as the anorexia disappears the mood of the child begins to change and a smile may be a good prognostic sign.

At this stage the treatment can be modified and will be similar for mild cases not requiring hospitalization–consisting of a more varied diet rich in protein. The mother's cooperation in the dietary regimen is important and should form an integral part of therapy, as her nutritional education is expanded.

NUTRITIONAL MARASMUS
Etiology and Epidemiology

Nutritional marasmus is common in nearly all developing countries and in contrast to kwashiorkor is more common in children under 1 year of age, although it is not restricted to this age group. The disease is a form of starvation and therefore the underlying causes are numerous but all involve lack of food and any kind of food. In the United States nutritional marasmus is occasionally seen in grossly neglected children, but may also occur secondary to such diseases as cystic fibrosis, celiac disease or overwhelming infections.

In developing countries a common cause is early cessation of breast feeding. This may be due to death of the mother, failure of lactation, separation of the infant from the mother, or most commonly the mother's desire to feed her infant from the bottle rather than the breast. In this latter event she may be influenced by advertisements and the impact of alien cultures into believing that this is a superior or more sophisticated method of infant feeding. Early cessation of breast feeding does not of course necessarily lead to marasmus. However, a large proportion of people in developing countries do not have sufficient income to purchase enough milk formula to feed a baby properly. As a result the tendency is to overdilute the mixture with water which then fails to provide adequate calories. Similarly few households in these countries have a safe water supply or items in their home which simplify the sterile preparation of bottles of formula for an infant. This combined with a lack of knowledge concerning hygiene commonly leads to the development of gastrointestinal infection which starts the vicious circle leading to marasmus.

Other common causes of marasmus are prematurity, mental deficiency and gastrointestinal disease such as diarrhea or malabsorption. Many of the factors listed under the etiology of kwashiorkor may also be involved.

The Disease

The following are the main features of nutritional marasmus:

(a) *Growth failure*–In all cases there is clear evidence of growth failure. If the age of the child is known the weight will be extremely low by normal standards and the height will also usually be below

Figure 5
Nutritional marasmus showing extreme wasting in child from Rotterdam, Holland, during World War II.

normal. In severe cases the loss of flesh is obvious. The ribs are prominent, the face has a characteristic monkey-like appearance, the limbs are very thin, but the abdomen may be protuberant and in general the child looks like the starved individual which he is.

(b) *Wasting*–The muscles are extremely wasted. There is little if any subcutaneous fat remaining. The skin hangs in wrinkles, especially around the buttocks and thighs.

(c) *Appetite*–Whereas the child with kwashiorkor has anorexia, the child with marasmus frequently has a good appetite. In fact, like any starving creature he may be ravenous, often sucking his hands and clothing.

(d) *Mental state*–Most children with marasmus appear bright eyed and alert. They are not usually disinterested or irritable, like children with kwashiorkor.

(e) *Anemia* is usually present.

(f) *Diarrhea* is common, but is not a constant feature.

An advanced case of nutritional marasmus presents an unmistakable picture. The infant is appallingly thin but the belly in contrast to the rest of the body may be protuberant. The disease, unlike kwashiorkor does not lead to edema or flaky paint dermatosis. Hair changes similar to kwashiorkor can occur, but are less common. Signs of vitamin deficiency, especially of vitamin A, may accompany marasmus.

Laboratory findings

Serum proteins may be reduced, but less so than in kwashiorkor.

The hydroxyproline-creatinine index[14] is low, but the ratio of essential to non-essential amino acids is less altered than in kwashiorkor.

The liver is not infiltrated with fat.

Treatment

Treatment is similar to that described for kwashiorkor, but an adequate intake of calories and protein is mandatory to allow for weight gain and growth.

14. Whitehead, R. G., *Lancet* 2:567, 1965.

Therefore, if dried skimmed milk is used as the basis for treatment, vegetable oil should be added to provide calories.

Anemia, infections, diarrhea and dehydration should be treated as described for kwashiorkor. In general, response to treatment in severe nutritional marasmus is slow and prolonged hospitalization is often necessary.

It is particularly important to ensure that the child is not discharged from treatment back to the very set of circumstances that led to the disease. Steps must be taken to insure that an adequate diet is provided for the child after it leaves the hospital.

CLINICAL FEATURES OF KWASHIORKOR AND MARASMUS COMPARED[15]

Clinical Feature	Kwashiorkor	Marasmus
Growth Failure	Present	Present
Edema	Present	Absent
Mental Changes	Present	Uncommon
Hepatomegaly	Common	Uncommon
Hair Changes	Common	Uncommon
Dermatosis (flaky paint)	Fairly Common	Absent
Anemia	Very Common	Common
Sub-Cutaneous Fat	Reduced but Present	Absent
Appetite	Poor	Good

15. Latham, M. C., adapted from *Human Nutrition in Tropical Africa*, FAO, Rome 1966.

MILD TO MODERATE PROTEIN-CALORIE MALNUTRITION

Although detailed descriptions have been given of kwashiorkor and nutritional marasmus it should be kept in mind that these are extreme clinical conditions in the wide spectrum which constitutes protein-calorie malnutrition. In hospital practice many intermediate forms will be encountered. More important however is the fact that for every clinical case of one of these diseases there are hundreds of children who have mild or moderate forms of protein-calorie malnutrition. From a public health point of view it is desirable to try to detect these mild cases and in some way to prevent them from becoming severe.

The best means of detecting mild degrees of protein-calorie malnutrition is to follow the growth and development of young children. A child who fails to grow normally is a candidate for severe protein-calorie malnutrition and the one factor which most frequently leads to a deterioration of nutritional status is an infectious disease.

Ideally, heights, weights and other parameters of development should be followed secularly in all children at risk. If this is not possible then growth failure indicated by low height or weight for age, forms a useful guide. There are at present no biochemical tests sufficiently developed which provide a better means of detecting early protein-calorie malnutrition than the measurement of height and weight.

A grading of malnutrition on the basis of weight for age is widely used in developing countries. This is the Gomez classification:[16]

Grade I Malnutrition—75 to 90% of expected weight for age

Grade II Malnutrition—60 to 75% of expected weight for age

Grade III Malnutrition—less than 60% of expected weight for age

Weight of course, can be lost very rapidly in a sick child or from gross dietary deficiencies. In contrast height once acquired cannot be lost except in aging adulthood. Height deficits therefore, provide a better indication of chronic malnutrition. However, height expressed as a percentage of normal height gives a false picture in that it indicates smaller deficits than does weight. It is better to state height age as a percentage of actual age.[17] For example, if the standard

16. Gomez, F., *J. Trop. Pediatrics* 2:77, 1956.
17. Latham, M. C., in *Calorie Deficiencies and Protein Deficiencies*, edited by McCance and Widdowson, J. and A. Churchill Ltd., London, 1968.

Figure 6
Malnutrition may be precipitated by infection. An unsanitary environment may lead to infectious disease and parasitosis.

age for reaching 84 cm. in height is 24 months then a child who is 84 cm. at age 36 months is 66 per cent of his height age.

Other anthropometric measures that have practical value include head circumference, chest circumference, upper arm circumference and skinfold thickness.[18]

MALNUTRITION AND SUBSEQUENT DEVELOPMENT

There is good scientific evidence to show that children who have suffered from protein-calorie malnutrition early in life have some permanent stunting of physical growth. Therefore, if the malnutrition has been prolonged serious dwarfing may result.

There is some evidence to suggest that protein-calorie malnutrition early in life may also result in failure of the child to reach his full potential of intellectual and psychological development.[19] In experimental animals it has been shown that behavioral abnormalities follow early malnutrition. It has also been found that baby rats malnourished during the suckling period subsequently have reduced numbers of cells in the brain.[20] This has been done by relating DNA to cell numbers.

A few studies have indicated that children who have had malnutrition early in life subsequently perform less well on a variety of mental tests than do children of the same age who have not had malnutrition. There are indications that malnourished children may never catch up to the other children in intelligence.[21] Some studies have also shown that the malnourished children also have reduced head circumference, a measure which may provide an indication of brain size.[22]

Research on the relationship of malnutrition to behavioral development is barely beginning. Therefore, although a definite association has been demonstrated between early protein-calorie malnutrition and subsequent poor intellectual perfomance it has not been proved that this relationship is one of cause and effect. Quite possibly some genetic and environmental factors which influence intellectual development of children may also be important in the etiology of malnutrition. Therefore, factors such as poverty, ignorant and illiterate parents, crowding, a high prevalence of infectious disease, poor learning opportunities and several others may be causes both of malnutrition and of poor psychological development in children.

NUTRITION AND INFECTION

In recent years the importance of the synergism of infection and dietary deficiencies in the causation of severe protein-calorie malnutrition has been realized.[23,24] The corollary is equally true, namely, that malnutrition is largely responsible for the increased severity and many of the devastating effects of infectious disease in malnourished children. Gastroenteritis, measles and other infections may frequently precipitate clinical malnutrition in a child. Similarly, diseases like measles which have a very low mortality in the well-nourished often have a high mortality in populations where malnutrition is prevalent.

Diarrheal disease in children at an age when they are being weaned from the breast is extremely common in developing countries and has been termed "weanling diarrhea." This is now commonly known to be a precipitating cause of malnutrition. It is also now clear that malnourished children more frequently develop diarrhea than do the well-nourished and that frequently the diarrhea may be due to malnutrition and not a pathogenic organism.

18. Jelliffe, D. B., *The Assessment of the Nutritional Status of the Community,* WHO, Geneva, 1966.
19. Cravioto, J., DeLicardie, E. R., and Birch, H. G., *Pediatrics, Suppl. 38*:369, 1966.
20. Winick, M. and Noble, A., *J. Nutr. 89*:300, 1966.
21. Monckeberg, F., in *Malnutrition, Learning and Behavior,* edited by Scrimshaw and Gordon, M.I.T. Press, Cambridge, 1968.
22. Stoch, M. B. and Smythe, P. M., *South African Med. J. 41*:1027, 1967.

23. *Nutrition and Infection,* World Health Organization Technical Reports Series No. 314, WHO, Geneva, 1965.
24. Scrimshaw, N. S., Taylor, C. E., and Gordon, J. E., *Am. J. Med. Sci. 237*: 367, 1959.

Xerophthalmia-Keratomalacia

Keratomalacia is a disease which is almost unknown in the United States, but is a common cause of blindness in some parts of the world, particularly in certain countries of Asia and the Middle East.[25] It is due to a dietary deficiency of vitamin A and occurs in young children and is often associated with protein-calorie malnutrition.

The Disease

An early sign of vitamin A deficiency is night blindness or the inability to see well in dim light. This is difficult to detect in young children. Vitamin A deficiency may also cause follicular hyperkeratosis of the skin and Bitot's spots of the eyes.

Xerophthalmia usually begins with a drying of the conjunctiva which loses its shining luster. This condition may then spread to the cornea which also becomes dull and loses its power to reflect. This pathological dryness of the eye, which robs it of its normal epithelial protection, is called xerophthalmia and is a precursor of keratomalacia.

If the condition remains untreated a necrotic process begins, followed by ulceration and leads to perforation, loss of intraocular fluid and a severe secondary infection may occur. The patient at this stage is often seriously ill with pyrexia and a grossly inflamed eye, and the patient is doomed to blindness in the afflicted eye.

If treatment is begun early or if food rich in vitamin A is consumed before the stage of perforation, then the ulcer may heal leaving perhaps only an opaque corneal scar. In some cases vascularization of the cornea precedes ulceration.

In vitamin A deficiency the concentration of vitamin A in the plasma is usually below 20 μg. per 100 ml. but may be so low as to be undetectable and it must be low for a prolonged period to produce clinical signs of vitamin A deficiency. Normal levels range from 30 to 50 μg. per 100 ml.

25. Oomen, H. A., McLaren, D. S., and Escapini, U., *Trop. Geograph. Med.* 16:271, 1964.

Figure 7a
Vitamin A Deficiency—Night Blindness is a useful and early diagnostic sign of vitamin A deficiency. The loss of visual acuity in dim light following exposure to bright light is illustrated.

Figure 7b
Both the normal individual and the vitamin A deficient subject see the headlights of an approaching car as shown in *Figure 7b*. After the car has passed the normal individual sees a wide stretch of road.

Figure 7c
The vitamin A-deficient subject can barely see a few feet ahead and cannot see the road sign at all.

Figure 8
Bitots spots—white foamy plaques on the temporal side of the cornea.

Figure 9
Xerophthalmia in an Indonesian child with severe involvement of one eye.

Figure 10
Keratomalacia in a young child.

Treatment

Severe cases of xerophthalmia should be treated as a medical emergency as the sight and life of the children is at stake. The recommended treatment is:

(a) Injection of a vitamin A preparation at an initial dose of 22.5 mg. (75,000 I.U.)

(b) 22.5 mg. (75,000 I.U.) vitamin A daily by mouth. This may be either a preparation of synthetic vitamin A or in the form of cod- or halibut-liver oil.

(c) Tetracycline or other antibiotic eye ointments should be instilled into both eyes every four hours for the first 48 hours and less frequently for the next 7 to 10 days.

(d) Riboflavin tablets 5 mg. three times daily.

(e) For a period of 7 to 10 days penicillin 600,000 units daily I.M. or some other antibiotic should be administered to combat secondary infection.

(f) A mixed diet, rich in vitamin A and carotene should be given.

(g) Protein-calorie malnutrition should be treated if present.

Thiamine Deficiency Syndromes Including Beriberi and the Wernicke-Korsakoff Syndrome

Beriberi

Beriberi is caused by a deficiency of the B vitamin thiamine, also known as B_1, when the ratio of its intake to the number of calories obtained from carbohydrate is low. The disease occurs predominantly among rice-eating peoples of the world because of the desire for refined or polished rice.

The Disease

There are various ways of dividing beriberi from a clinical viewpoint. Here it will be grouped into three forms: (1) Wet beriberi, (2) Dry beriberi, and (3) Infantile beriberi. These three clinical forms of the disease have many different features and yet appear to be caused by the same dietary deficiency and occur in the same endemic areas.

Early clinical features common to both
wet and dry beriberi

Both wet and dry beriberi usually begin in a similar mild way. The person tires easily, his limbs feel heavy and weak and he may get a mild degree of swelling around the ankles. There may be a numbness and a feeling of "pins and needles" in the legs, as well as occasional palpitations of the heart.

Examination at this stage might reveal some reduced motor power, perhaps a slight alteration in gait and a patchy anesthesia over the skin of the lower legs. The rice eater in the orient or the alcoholic elsewhere will often continue his normal activities and not seek early medical advice. The condition at this stage would improve with a better diet or with thiamine administration. Left untreated, the condition might remain almost static for months but at any stage might progress to either clinical wet or dry beriberi.

Wet beriberi

The name wet beriberi is used because the main feature of the disease is the accumulation of edema fluid in the legs and often in the scrotum, face and trunk. The patient frequently develops cardiac palpitations, chest pain and later dyspnea. The pulse is rapid and often irregular. The neck veins are distended with visible pulsations and the heart becomes enlarged. The volume of urine tends to be diminished but despite the edema contains no albumin. This latter is an important diagnostic feature.

A patient with wet beriberi is in danger of rapid deterioration, acute circulatory failure, and death.

Dry beriberi

This is termed dry because edema is not a feature. The condition is really neuritic beriberi and is similar to peripheral neuritis due to other causes.

Anesthesia and paresthesia of the feet followed by increased difficulty in walking is a common feature. On examination the patient has a peculiar ataxic gait, foot drop and wrist drop are common, there is considerable muscular wasting, there are anesthetic patches especially over the tibia and there is tenderness of the calves and other muscles when pressure is applied. The sufferer has great difficulty in rising from the squatting position.

The disease is often chronic, and at any stage improvement may slowly occur if the subject consumes a better diet or receives treatment with thiamine. Untreated the disease progresses, the patient eventually becomes bed ridden and frequently dies of some chronic infection.

Infantile beriberi

This is the only important dietary deficiency disease which occurs in otherwise normal infants under six months of age who are receiving adequate quantities of breast milk. It is due to inadequate thiamine in the milk of a lactating mother whose diet is deficient in this vitamin. The mother may however, have no overt signs of beriberi.

Infantile beriberi commonly occurs between 2 and 6 months of age. In the acute form the infant develops dyspnea and cyanosis and dies of cardiac failure with unnerving rapidity. In chronic forms, the classical sign is aphonia, the infant going through the motions of crying like a well rehearsed mime, but without emitting much of any sound. The infant is thin and wasted, diarrhea and vomiting may develop and due to a deficiency of calories and other nutrients the infant becomes marasmic. Edema occasionally is seen and convulsions may occur in the terminal stages.

Diagnosis of wet, dry and infantile beriberi

Diagnosis may be difficult when only the early manifestations are present. A history of a diet deficient in thiamine and improvement on a good diet or following treatment with thiamine will help to establish the diagnosis.

Figure 11
Edema in beriberi.

Wet beriberi must be distinguished from renal edema and congestive cardiac failure. In both these latter conditions there is albuminuria; in beriberi there is not.

Measurement of blood levels of thiamine and thiamine phosphate is of limited value. More useful are determinations of blood lactate and blood pyruvate levels especially if performed after glucose administration and exercise. Urinary excretion of thiamine per gram of creatinine provides a good index of thiamine intake but is useful for surveys rather than for diagnosis in the individual patient.

Treatment

Wet beriberi

(a) Absolute bed rest.

(b) Thiamine 10 to 20 mg. daily by injection. When clinical improvement is evident replace injections with oral thiamine 10 mg. daily.

(c) Full nutritious diet rich in B vitamins but low in carbohydrate.

Severe wet beriberi is a very gratifying disease to treat for the response is usually dramatic. Diuresis and rapid reduction of dyspnea occur with elimination of edema in a few days.

Dry beriberi

(a) Rest in bed.

(b) Thiamine 10 mg. daily by mouth.

(c) Nutritious diet including B complex vitamins.

(d) Physiotherapy.

Improvement is often very slow.

Infantile beriberi

(a) Immediate injection of thiamine 5 mg. and daily injections for four days.

(b) Thiamine 10 mg. orally twice a day to the mother if the child is being breast fed.

(c) Nutritious and thiamine-rich diet to both mother and child.

Thiamine deficiency in the U.S.

Although classical beriberi is uncommon in the U.S., thiamine deficiency is by no means a rarity. It is confined mainly to the alcoholic population. Alcoholism is an increasingly prevalent condition and several clinical features previously believed to be due to chronic alcoholic intoxication are now known to be the result of nutritional deficiencies.

Wernicke-Korsakoff Syndrome

Wernicke's disease is characterized by eye signs (nystagmus, diplopia, paralysis of the externi recti muscles and sometimes ophthalmoplegia), ataxia and mental changes. Korsakoff's psychosis leads to a loss of memory of the immediate past and often an elaborate confabulation which tends to conceal this amnesia.

It is now generally agreed that any distinction between Wernicke's disease and Korsakoff's psychosis may be artificial in the alcoholic patient. Korsakoff's psychosis may be regarded as the psychotic component of Wernicke's disease.[26]

This view is supported by the fact that many patients who appear with ocular palsy, ataxia and confusion and who survive, later show the amnestic disorder of Korsakoff's psychosis. Similarly patients in mental institutions with Korsakoff's psychosis often show the stigmata of Wernicke's disease even years after the illness. Pathological evidence also indicates the unity of the two conditions.

Proof that the Wernicke-Korsakoff syndrome is due to thiamine deficiency and not to chronic alcohol intoxication is shown by the fact that the condition responds to thiamine alone, even if the individual continues to consume alcohol.

Of overriding importance in this syndrome is the fact that irreversible brain damage ensues rapidly and therefore early recognition and treatment are vital. If there is any suspicion that a patient may have this condition, he should immediately receive 5 to 10 mg. of thiamine by injection even before a definitive diagnosis is made.

Prevention

The prevention of the Wernicke-Korsakoff syn-

drome calls for considerable public health ingenuity. Possibilities suggested[27] have included:

(a) The "immunization" of alcoholics with large doses of thiamine at regular intervals. The development of a suitable depot carrier to reduce the frequency of these injections would be very helpful.

(b) The fortification of alcoholic beverages with thiamine.

(c) A provision by public health authorities that thiamine impregnated snacks be available on bar counters.

The cost of any of these measures would almost certainly be less than is the present enormous expenditure on institutional care of those who have suffered from Wernicke-Korsakoff disease.

Other thiamine deficiency states

Alcoholic polyneuropathy, a condition similar to neuritic beriberi, is also a disease due to a dietary deficiency of thiamine.

An optic or retrobulbar neuritis which occurred in prison camps in World War II was probably due to thiamine deficiency. This condition, also known as nutritional amblyopia was at least in part due to thiamine deficiency.

Pellagra

Pellagra which used to be common in the southern United States is now seldom seen in this country. The disease is associated with a corn (maize) diet and is primarily due to a dietary deficiency of niacin. Although corn has more niacin than some other staple foods it seems that this is not all utilized, most likely because it is in a bound form unavailable to the body. The human body can convert the amino acid tryptophan into niacin and so a high-protein diet rich in tryptophan will help prevent pellagra. The main protein in corn is zein which is very low in tryptophan content.

26. Victor, M. and Adams, R. D., *Am. J. Clin. Nutr.* 9:379, 1961.

27. Latham, M. C., in *Present Knowledge in Nutrition*, The Nutrition Foundation, Inc., New York 1967.

Casal's Necklace—Advanced Pellagra. Dermatitis outlining the exposed area of the neck is pathognomonic of pellagra, as are the characteristic lesions on the backs of the hands. Either sunlight or heat from a stove may have been the precipitating factor.

The Disease

Pellagra to the medical student is portrayed by the four D's— dermatitis, diarrhea, dementia, and death. The disease is most often diagnosed from the characteristic appearance of the skin lesions. These lesions are often symmetrical in appearance and occur on areas of the body exposed to sunlight such as the face, the neck and the forearms. In Caucasians the skin lesions at first resemble the erythema of sunburn. In Negroes there is a hyperpigmentation. The affected areas become dry, scaly and cracked and if the condition progresses desquamation commonly occurs. There may be cracking and fissuring, and occasionally the skin becomes blistered. In persons wearing an open-neck shirt, the upper chest and lower neck are affected and this lesion is known as Casal's necklace.

Digestive symptoms include abdominal pain and diarrhea. Frequently the tongue and mouth are sore, and sometimes angular stomatitis and cheilosis, usually associated with riboflavin deficiency, occur. The tongue is often red, smooth and raw looking.

Involvement of the nervous system manifests itself by extremely variable symptoms and signs. The commonest of these are irritability, loss of memory, insomnia and anxiety. These may lead to dementia. It used to be common for persons to be incarcerated in mental institutions without anyone realizing that the mental condition was due to pellagra. In areas where corn is the primary staple food all persons admitted to mental institutions should be examined for evidence of pellagra.

Mild sensory and motor changes occasionally occur in pellagra, but paralysis is very rare.

Diagnosis

Diagnosis is usually made on the basis of the dietary history and on physical examination.

Treatment

Hospital admission is only necessary for very serious cases. Niacinamide 50 to 100 mg. three times daily by intramuscular injection for the first 3-4 days

Figure 12b
Same patient after
nicotinamide therapy.

Figure 13a   Figure 13b

Glossitis is the earliest diagnostic sign of pellagra brought about by nicotinamide deficiency. It starts with a burning sensation, which is followed either by edema or by desquamation of the epithelium. Dental indentations (Figure 13a) result from edema. Tip and margins of tongue are made scarlet red and shiny by desquamation of the epithelium (Figure 13b). There are signs of healed angular stomatitis, indicating a previous riboflavin deficiency.

Figure 14
Infant with scurvy in the "Pithed Frog" position. Because movement is painful, the scorbutic infant usually lies on its back and makes little attempt to lift the leg or arm that hurts. Both legs may be tender, and sometimes both arms as well. This is usually the first sign of scurvy.

and subsequently by mouth should form the basis of treatment. A daily diet of high caloric value and containing at least 100 grams of good quality protein is recommended.

If abdominal burning or diarrhea are troublesome, an easily digestable diet low in fiber content should be given. Sedation with barbiturates is recommended for the first few days of treatment. Those with mental disturbances benefit greatly from a tranquilizer prescribed in relatively large doses. A vitamin B complex preparation is useful to counteract concurrent deficiencies of other B vitamins.

Scurvy

Today scurvy is a rare disease. It results from a deficiency of vitamin C and usually occurs only after a considerable time in persons on a diet containing very little fresh food. Daily intakes of vitamin C very much below the recommended allowances, even for periods of several months, usually do not result in scurvy.

Vitamin C is necessary for the formation and healthy upkeep of intercellular material. In scurvy the walls of the capillaries lack solidity and become fragile resulting in hemorrhage from various sites.

The Disease
The following symptoms and signs may occur:

(a) Tenderness of the extremities, muscle weakness and suppressed appetite.

(b) Gums become swollen and bleed easily; teeth may become loose.

(c) Hemorrhages of a petechial type often occur in the skin.

(d) Hemorrhages in other areas may manifest themselves as nose bleeds, hematuria, melena, splinter hemorrhages below the nails and painful sub-periosteal hemorrhages.

(e) Delayed healing of wounds and heightened risk of infection.

(f) Anemia and shortness of breath.

A patient with scurvy and some of the above symptoms and signs, though not appearing very seriously ill, may suddenly collapse and die of cardiac failure.

Infantile scurvy (Barlow's disease)

Infantile scurvy usually occurs in infants, 2 to 12 months of age, who are bottle fed with a milk formula to which vitamin C has not been added and who do not receive any other source of vitamin C. The vitamin C in milk is destroyed by heat in the pasteurization or drying of milk.

The infant with scurvy cries when the limbs are touched or moved due to pain and tenderness. The infant often lies with his limbs placed in what has been called the "pithed frog" position. Swellings due to hemorrhages may be felt especially in the legs and there may be obvious bruising of the body. Hemorrhages may occur from any of the sites mentioned previously for adult scurvy but gum bleeding does not occur unless there are erupted teeth.

Diagnosis of Scurvy

The capillary fragility test is useful but there are other conditions beside scurvy which influence capillary strength. Estimations of ascorbic acid in serum, or preferably in white blood cells, may be useful. If serum ascorbic acid is present, the disease is not scurvy. Decreased urinary excretion of ascorbic acid is an early sign. Radiographs aid in the diagnosis of infantile scurvy and in older subjects "scurvy lines" of the tibia and femur are helpful in the diagnosis.

The concentration of ascorbic acid in the blood plasma reflects the dietary intake and does not indicate the degree of depletion of the bodily stores. It is better to measure the concentration of ascorbic acid in the leukocytes. Levels below 2 mg./100 ml. provide presumptive evidence of scurvy.

Treatment

Because of the danger of sudden death, even in the patient who looks reasonably well, there is a need for immediate vigorous treatment. It is advisable to give by mouth a loading dose of 1000 mg. ascorbic acid followed by 250 mg. four times daily for 6 to 7 days when the dosage can usually be reduced to 50 mg. twice a day until recovery is complete. The patient should also be put on a diet containing plenty of fresh fruit and vegetables. Ascorbic acid by injection is necessary if the patient is vomiting and is useful for the treatment of infants.

Rickets and Osteomalacia

In both rickets and osteomalacia there is a lack of calcium retention in the skeleton. The conditions are, however, due mainly to a deficiency of vitamin D and not of dietary calcium. Vitamin D is obtained both from the diet and from exposure of the skin to sunlight. The average unsupplemented diet contains only relatively small amounts of vitamin D but nowadays this vitamin is added to many processed foods, especially those commonly consumed by young children. Vitamin D deficiency is therefore uncommon in children and is very rare in adults in the United States.

RICKETS
The Disease

Unlike many other deficiency diseases the child with rickets often has the superficial appearance of being plump and well fed. This frequently gives the mother a false sense of security. The story has often been told of the rachitic child winning the baby show because it appeared so fat and well nourished. The child, however, tends to be miserable and closer examination will reveal the flabby toneless state of the muscles. Another feature is the general impairment of normal development. The child is frequently late in reaching all the milestones in his early life. He is slow to learn to sit, to walk and to get his teeth. Other generalized signs include gastrointestinal upsets and excessive sweating of the head.

Figure 16a
7-10-35, Roentgenologic Findings (Right and Left Legs and Ankles). X-ray films of the legs and ankles show a marked flaring and widening of the diaphysis above the epiphyseal line. The zone between the shaft and epiphysis is increased in thickness with ragged fringy margins. There is a marked bowing of the lower end of tibia.   Conclusion–Rachitic infant

Figure 15
Two Girls with Rickets: The cases of Ethel and Evelyn
These patients, twins, were first seen on July 10, two days after they had won first prize at a baby show. Both infants were female and appeared to be well nourished. They were markedly obese. On physical examination, there was a definite craniotabes. The anterior fontanelle was open. There was a flaring of the lower rib margin and a well marked rachitic rosary. There was an extreme bowing of both legs, which was more marked in the lower third. "X-ray films of the legs and ankles showed a marked flaring and widening of the diaphesis above the epiphyseal line. The zone between the shaft and the epihysis is increased in thickness with ragged, fringy margins. There is a marked bowing of the lower end of the tibia."   Diagnosis—Rachitic infant

These children had been raised on artificial feeding with no supplemental vitamin D. They were placed on high doses of vitamin D concentrate. A very rapid improvement was noted in both cases, especially that of Ethel, whose condition was so severe that she was placed in bed with traction on both feet. We were not able to secure X-ray films again until February 7. At this time there was an increase in the density of the bone with a marked thickening of the cortex of the shaft on the concave side. The epiphyseal line is much narrower and the margin is much more regular in outline.

Figure 16b
2-7-36, Roentgenologic Findings (Right and Left Legs and Ankles). X-ray films after treatment show an increase in the density of the bone. There is a marked thickening of the cortex of the shaft on the concave side. The epiphyseal line is much narrower and the margin is much more regular in outline.

Conclusion–X-ray films show a marked improvement.

Figure 17a
Child from moderately well-to-do family with marked bow legs
due to rickets.

The main signs of the disease and those on which
the diagnosis of rickets is made are the skeletal
changes. One early feature is a swelling of the epiphysis of the long bones. This may first be found at
the wrist where the radius is affected. Another classical site is at the costo-chondral junctions where swellings occur. This produces a bead-like appearance
which has received the name "rachitic rosary." Deformities of the chest lead to the formation of Harri-
son's sulcus and pigeon breast. Swellings of the epiphyses of the tibia, fibula and femur may also be
seen.

In young infants craniotabes is often the first sign
of rickets. This consists of areas of softening of the
skull usually affecting the occipital and parietal
bones. There is also delayed closing of the anterior
fontanel. In severe rickets there may be bossing of
the skull.

When a child with rickets begins to stand and walk
he often develops new deformities due to the soft,
weak character of the bones. The commonest of these
are bowlegs and less frequently knock-knees. More
serious, however, are deformities of the spine leading
to kyphosis. Changes in the pelvis though often not
obvious may subsequently result in difficulty in childbirth in women who have had rickets during childhood.

Tetany due to a reduction in the level of serum calcium sometimes occurs. It presents an unmistakable
picture with spasm of the hands; the thumb being
drawn into the palm.

Diagnosis

X-ray examination will reveal abnormalities and is
also helpful in showing progress during treatment.
Radiographs, especially of the wrists but also of the
ends of long bones at other sites are useful in diagnosis. This will usually reveal characteristic changes
in the epiphyses. The outline of the joint is blurred,
the epiphyseal line is broadened and later the end of
the bone shaft appears saucered. The trabeculation of

Figure 17b
Back view of same child.

Figure 17c
Close-up from back, note angle of feet.

the bone becomes coarse and there is a decrease in bone density. Curvature of the bones may be even more evident in radiographs than is found in clinical examination, especially in a plump child. Some of the early radiographic changes in rickets are rather similar to those of infantile scurvy.

The serum alkaline phosphatase is usually elevated well above the normal range of 5-15 Bodansky units. A level above 20 units in a child is very suggestive of rickets. The serum phosphorus is usually reduced to 2-4 mg./100 ml. (normal = 4.5-5.5 mg./100 ml.), but the serum calcium is frequently normal or only slightly reduced, being around 10 mg./100 ml.

Treatment

The basis of treatment is the provision of adequate quantities of vitamin D at the same time ensuring an adequate intake of calcium. Vitamin preparations that provide about 75 μg. (3000 I.U.) of vitamin D daily is the recommended therapy. Calcium supplementation is usually given as milk.

Simultaneously with treatment the mother should be educated regarding the value of sunshine on the body as well as given good nutritional instruction.

Mild bony deformities tend to right themselves following dietary treatment, but in more serious cases some degree of deformity may persist.

Osteomalacia

Osteomalacia is the adult counterpart of rickets and has the same general causes. It occurs much more frequently in women than in men. It is most common in women on a poor diet who have been depleted of calcium by many years of pregnancies and lactation, who get very little vitamin D in their diet and who are protected from the sun by their clothing and confinement indoors. The condition is usually very rare in the U.S.

The Disease

Pain occurs in the bones of the pelvis, lower back and the legs. Tenderness may be elicited by pressure

Figure 18a
Rickets in a 3-month-old infant.

Figure 18b
Healing after 28 days of vitamin D treatment.

Figure 18c
After 41 days. In these photographs no shadow is cast by the epiphyses, which are still unossified.

Rickets is recognized by X-ray most readily in the wrist. The uncalcified lower ends of the bones are porous, ragged, and saucer-shaped.

on the affected bones. Deformities occur later, especially in the pelvis and spine. The patient may walk with his feet widely spaced and may appear to waddle. Spontaneous fractures often are a complication of severe osteomalacia. In some cases tetany develops and may be seen as involuntary twitchings of the muscles of the face and by carpopedal spasms.

Diagnosis

Radiographs will show extensive demineralization, bony deformities and if present, fractures. The level of serum alkaline phosphatase is raised above the maximum normal adult level of 5 Bodansky units and the concentration of serum calcium often decreases below 8 mg./100 ml.

Treatment

Vitamin D, 125 μg. (50,000 I.U.) daily should be given as a vitamin preparation. Calcium is easily provided as milk if available; otherwise some other form such as calcium lactate is adequate. Freedom of the exposed skin to sunlight should be encouraged. Good obstetrical care is very important in women who have pelvic abnormalities due to osteomalacia.

Endemic Goiter

Goiter is the name used for any swelling of the thyroid gland. When it occurs sporadically it may be due to a number of different causes not related to diet and not, therefore, relevant to this monograph. However, where goiter is common or endemic in a district or in a community, the cause is usually nutritional, due to a lack of the mineral nutrient iodine.

In endemic goiter areas, frequently many people have some enlargement of the thyroid gland and a smaller number have large and obvious swellings of the neck. By far the commonest cause of endemic goiter is a deficiency of iodine in the diet of those affected. The amount of iodine present in soil varies from place to place and this affects the quantity both in food grown and in the water supply of the area.

Sea foods such as fish, shellfish and seaweed are rich sources of iodine. Endemic goiter areas are usually far from the sea.

It has been found in experimental animals that there are certain foods which if eaten in large quantities, make the animal more liable to develop goiter even if normal quantities of iodine are consumed. Substances which have this effect are called goitrogens and are known to exist in certain varieties of cabbage, kale, turnips and some other vegetables. There is little evidence to incriminate dietary goitrogens as being important in endemic goiter in man.

In the U.S.A. endemic areas of goiter are mainly in the states bordering on Canada, especially the Great Lakes area and those between the Rocky Mountains and the Appalachians.

Physiology of endemic goiter

The thyroid gland requires iodine to produce thyroxine which contains 64 per cent iodine. When iodine is deficient the gland enlarges to try to compensate for this difficulty in producing thyroxine. This basically is the mechanism at work in goiter due to iodine deficiency.

The normal thyroid gland contains about 8 milligrams of iodine and this may be reduced to 1 to 2 milligrams in persons with goiter. The thyroid gland is under the control of the anterior pituitary gland. Iodine is absorbed from the intestines at a rate which is dependent on thyroid activity. The rate of secretion of thyroid stimulating hormone (T.S.H.) by the anterior pituitary depends upon the concentration of thyroid hormones circulating in the blood. Thyroxine administration will therefore inhibit T.S.H. secretion.

The iodine uptake in normal persons is proportional to the blood concentration of the thyroid hormones. It has been shown that the uptake of radioactive iodine is increased in hyperthyroidism and decreased in hypothyroidism. There are, however, other factors which can influence it.

The total iodine content in whole blood is usually $10 \mu g. \pm 4 \mu g.$ of which $6 \mu g. \pm 2 \mu g.$ is protein-bound. The protein-bound iodine (PBI) is reduced in hypothyroidism and elevated in hyperthyroidism. The amount of iodine in the urine is dependent mainly on the iodine intake in the diet and on thyroid activity.

Endemic goiter is diagnosed when there is thyroid enlargement in a patient living in an area where endemic goiter is known to occur, where there is evidence that the iodine intake of the patient is low and where other causes of thyroid enlargement can be ruled out.

Urinary excretion of iodine in these individuals would usually be below 100 $\mu g.$ daily, the protein-bound iodine is in the normal range and the uptake of radioactive I^{131} is often increased.

Goiter surveys

When investigating goiter prevalence in a population the thyroid gland of a representative sample should be examined both visually and by palpation in order to estimate the degree of enlargement. Each lobe of the normal thyroid gland is about the size of the thumb nail of the person being examined. A useful classification of goiter size is that suggested by W.H.O.[28] which can be summarized as follows:

Group 0–Persons without goiter and persons with the thyroid less than five times enlarged.

Group 1–Persons with the thyroid more than five times enlarged but not easily visible with the head in normal position.

Group 2–Persons with goiters which are easily visible with the head in normal position, but which are smaller than Group 3.

Group 3–Persons with large goiters which can be easily recognized at a considerable distance and which may be disfiguring.

The Disease

Goiter is more common in females particularly at puberty and during pregnancy. The enlargement of

28. *Endemic Goiter,* World Health Organization Monograph Series No. 4, WHO, Geneva, 1960.

Figure 19
Drawing of types of goiter.

Classification of Goiters
Neck profiles illustrating categories of thyroid enlargement

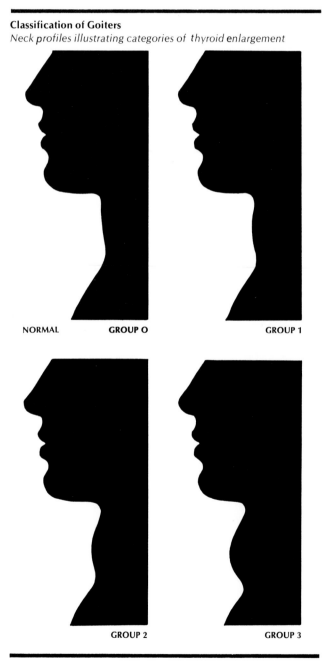

NORMAL   GROUP O   GROUP 1

GROUP 2   GROUP 3

the gland may be smooth and is then said to be a colloid goiter or it may be lumpy and is then called an adenomatous or nodular goiter.

Endemic goiter, in which there is a benign enlargement of the thyroid gland, may cause no symptoms. The enlargement is merely evidence of a deficient intake of iodine. Appropriate treatment will prevent both further enlargement and the complications which may accompany goiter and in many cases will cause the gland to return to its normal size. Untreated, the gland may enlarge to a size which is obvious and presents a cosmetic problem. Further enlargement may produce pressure symptoms such as difficulty in breathing, persistent cough or voice changes. A person with a simple goiter may develop the symptoms and signs of hyperthyroidism. Carcinoma of the thyroid is more common in those with goiter.

Cretinism in children occurs most commonly in endemic goiter areas and is usually due to severe iodine deficiency of the mother. The infant might appear normal at birth, but is slow to develop, small in size, mentally dull, has a thick skin and a characteristic face with depressed nose and often a protruding, enlarged tongue. Deaf mutism and mental retardation are found more frequently in the children of mothers with enlarged thyroid glands.

Treatment

Small diffuse colloid goiters will reduce in size and may disappear with suitable iodine therapy or with an increased dietary intake of iodine. The recommended treatment is Lugol's solution of iodine 0.5 ml. per day by mouth in water.

More dramatic improvement, especially in those with larger goiters, can be achieved by the use of thyroid extract or thyroxine. If this form of therapy is used, the weight, pulse rate and if possible the basal metabolic rate of the patient should be checked at regular intervals. Treatment should start with a small dose; e.g., thyroid extract ½ gr. daily and be increased gradually to 2 gr. daily. Weight loss, increased pulse rate and a raised BMR are indications of hyperthyroidism and are a signal to reduce the dosage.

Surgical treatment consisting of sub-total thyroidectomy is indicated for large goiters, especially the adenomatous type and for those exceptional cases that do not respond to iodine or thyroid extract.

Prevention of endemic goiter

Where goiter is prevalent it constitutes a public health problem and should be tackled as such. The most satisfactory measure is the addition of iodide to all salt sold in the area. This will reduce the size of many existing goiters ad will prevent most goiters from developing in the future.

Salt is most commonly iodized with sodium or potassium iodide to a level which provides about 0.5 grams of iodine to 1 kilogram of salt. The less volatile potassium iodate is preferable to iodide for iodination in hot, humid countries or regions. When endemic goiter is a problem it is desirable to pass legislation to ensure that all salt is iodized. Unfortunately legislation does not now exist throughout the U.S. or in most states to require the iodinization of all table salt or salt used in processed foods. Iodized and non-iodized salt is available in stores, displayed side by side, and there is recent evidence of increasing iodine deficiency in the U.S. This is really inexcusable.

Figure 20
Goiter in a young woman.

Figure 21
Advanced nodular goiters in an endemic area in Tanzania.

Nutrients

Protein

Dietary proteins furnish the necessary sources of amino acids and nitrogen for synthesis of body proteins and the array of other nitrogen-containing compounds excepting the nitrogen-containing vitamins. Most of the dietary protein is utilized as amino acids and absorbed by the intestinal mucosa after hydrolysis of complex peptide chains. Some twenty-two amino acids are of biological importance. Of these, eight so-called essential amino acids cannot be synthesized by man in amounts necessary for his needs.[29] These are lysine, leucine, isoleucine, methionine, phenylalanine, threonine, tryptophan, and valine. In addition, an exogenous supply of histidine is necessary for early growth and development. Requirements for the other amino acids are met either through exogenous sources or endogenous sources through synthesis from appropriate metabolic precursors and exogenous amino nitrogen.

Dietary proteins are supplied by both animal and plant materials. The nutritional quality of proteins from various sources is a function of the particular amino acids they contain in relation to essential amino acid requirements.

In general, protein from animal sources is of greater nutritional value because it contains all of the essential amino acids plus the non-essential ones. Proteins from cereals and vegetables are relatively deficient in certain amino acids, particularly lysine, tryptophan, threonine and methionine, depending on the specific cereal or vegetable and in addition provide less of all the *essential* amino acids per unit weight of protein than do those from animal sources. On the other hand, relatively small amounts of a high quality animal protein can efficiently supplement the relative amino acid deficiencies in diets obtained mainly from plant protein. Similarly appropriate mixtures of cereals, legumes or other vegetable foods may have a protein quality approaching that of animal foods.

In adults there is little if any absorption of peptide chains. The amino acids themselves are absorbed by an active transport system against a concentration gradient. Specificities in the transfer sites lead to differential rates of absorption and to competition in the transport of amino acids across the intestinal mucosa. A similar transfer system operates in other cells as well. There is no known "pool"—in the usual metabolic sense—of amino acids. And so a continuing, normal level of protein synthesis requires the continuous availability of the entire array of necessary amino acids. The removal of even one essential amino acid from the diet leads rather rapidly to a lower level of protein synthesis in the body.

Minimal protein requirements for a healthy adult represent the sum of the requirements for the essential amino acids plus sufficient utilizable nitrogen to maintain overall synthesis of nitrogen containing molecules. Nitrogen loss occurs in the urine, the feces, the skin, hair, and nails. Though there are considerable problems in measuring minimal protein requirement, it is of the order of 0.3 to 0.4 gm. protein/kg./day, assuming a reasonable amount of high quality protein or an appropriate mixture of cereal or vegetable protein with an adequate level of overall calories. With lower quality proteins, greater quantities are required to maintain nitrogen balance. Early growth and development, pregnancy, lactation, and periods of physical stress add to the basal requirement for protein. Recommended allowances include a two-to-three-fold "safety factor" over minimal requirements and apply to the ranges of quality in mixed proteins ordinarily consumed.

It is the very high (on a body weight basis) requirement for protein during early growth and development which makes this age group especially vulnerable to dietary deprivation.

In addition, the sometimes very marked degradation of protein and excretion of urinary nitrogen which accompanies the stress of even ordinarily mild childhood illnesses, puts such an added burden on an

29. Rose, W. C., *Federation Proc.* 8:546, 1949.

already tenuously nourished infant that it can start the spiral to frank, clinical malnutrition.

Carbohydrate

Carbohydrates comprise the major energy source for populations throughout the world and, being derived from foods readily and efficiently grown in nearly all climates, are cheaper than animal proteins and fats. The carbohydrate contribution to total daily calories is about 45% in the diets of people in highly developed areas. Whereas for the $7/8$ of the world's population that rely mainly on plants as sources of food, this contribution amounts to about 70% and may be as high as 90%.

The common hexoses—glucose, fructose, galactose, and mannose—are the digestion products absorbed from the gastrointestinal hydrolysis of the di- and polysaccharides occuring in foods.

In affluent societies half to two-thirds of the carbohydrate is furnished by starches, about a quarter by sucrose, and the rest is provided by lactose, glucose, fructose, and partly digestible polysaccharides. Refined sugar, by which is generally meant sucrose, provides in adult diets about 25% of the total carbohydrate or only 10 to 15% of the total daily calories. In the diets of children, sucrose is generally more prevalent, approaching half of the total carbohydrate or 20 to 25% of the total calories. In lesser developed areas the types of carbohydrate are different. Sucrose and lactose are consumed in smaller quanties, while starches make up most of the carbohydrate. A trend in American diets is the decreasing consumption of starches. Per capita consumption of sucrose has been quite constant. Cereals and vegetables contribute to the vitamin and mineral intake where they provide the major source of calories. In American diets the increased use of refined carbohydrates may produce constraints on the achievement of adequate nutrient intakes in very low-calorie diets.

There are no specific requirements established for carbohydrates as to type, source or amount. During starvation and with calorie restricted diets, carbohydrates serve to spare body proteins for energy purposes; as little as 100 gm. per day (400 calories) of carbohydrates can prevent the water and electrolyte loss attendant with protein catabolism, and probably as little as 40 gm. per day will prevent the development of ketosis.

Fats

Fats and oils in nutrition have historically been associated with the energy or caloric value of a diet and with its satiety value. This is because they provide twice as many calories per unit of weight as either carbohydrate or protein (9 Calories per gram versus 4) and because most people enjoy the taste of fats as they are characteristically used in our diets. Because fats remain in the stomach appreciably longer than carbohydrates or proteins, they tend to give a feel of "gastronomic satisfaction" for a somewhat longer period of time. More recently the interest in fats has been less on their caloric and satiety properties and more on their influence on the level of cholesterol in the blood and their association with atherosclerosis.

About 98% of dietary fats are triglycerides or compounds of glycerol and specific fatty acids. Since glycerol has three hydroxyl groups, each of which can combine with a fatty acid, we speak of triglycerides, diglycerides, and monoglycerides depending upon how many of the hydroxyl groups of the glycerol molecule have been esterified with a fatty acid. Additionally these fatty acids may be saturated, monounsaturated, or polyunsaturated. The term "saturation" refers to the degree of hydrogenation of the carbon atoms of the fatty acid chain. When the maximum number of hydrogen atoms are attached to the carbon atoms of the fatty acid chain, the chain is "saturated" with hydrogen–a saturated fat. If the carbon chain has one double bond and hence can accept two more hydrogen atoms, we call the fat monounsaturated. If the carbon chain has two or more double bonds and thus can accept four or more hydrogen atoms, we call the fat polyunsaturated. As previously stated all naturally occurring fats are mixtures of saturated, monounsaturated, and polyunsaturated fats, but the mixtures vary widely in composition. Thus, butter averages 66% saturates, 31% monounsaturates, and 3% polyunsaturates. Soybean oil averages 15% saturates, 25% monounsaturates, and 60% polyunsaturates while safflower oil has a still higher percentage of polyunsaturates, approximately 75% and correspondingly lower amount of monounsaturates and saturates.

In the processes of digestion, fats are mostly hydrolyzed into di- and monoglycerides and fatty acids by the action of various enzymes–lipases. As these lipases are present in pancreatic and intestinal juices, most of the digestion of fat takes place in the upper part of the small intestine. In the small intestine the fats are emulsified by the bile and this process facilitates the enzymatic action of the various lipases. Ordinarily most 12-carbon and longer fatty acids upon being emulsified and hydrolyzed, are absorbed into the lymphatic system and transported in association with cholesterol, phospholipids, and protein; these particles are termed chylomicrons. The chylomicrons then undergo a process of dissolution brought about by the action of an enzyme, lipoprotein lipase, found in blood and tissue.

In recent years finely divided and stable emulsions of fat have been prepared which may be given intravenously. Such emulsions are metabolized similarly to fat which has been eaten and they serve a useful role when complete intravenous nutrition is necessary for periods of several weeks.

Because the level of cholesterol in the blood is one of the factors associated with the development of coronary heart disease and other manifestations of atherosclerosis, and as the type of dietary fat is an important factor influencing the level of cholesterol in the blood, interest in fat has greatly increased in recent years. In general, the saturated fats increase the level of blood cholesterol, the monounsaturated fats have no effect, and the polyunsaturated fats decrease the cholesterol level. There is as yet no clear biochemical explanation for these regulating effects.

The common saturated fats of our diet are meat fat, milk fat, butter, cream, most cheese and coconut oil. Olive and peanut oils are examples of oils in which the predominant fats are monounsaturated. Soya, corn, cottonseed and safflower oils are the common oils in which the predominant fat is polyunsaturated because of the linoleic acid they contain. A diet designed to lower the level of cholesterol in the blood is low in saturated fat and high in polyunsaturated fat (see Section on Cardiovascular Disease).

The four commonly used polyunsaturated vegetable oils average 50% or more linoleic acid (safflower oil is 70% linoleic acid). In the preparation of these oils for commercial use in products such as shortenings and margarine and to give the oils greater stability, they are partially hydrogenated. This, of course, reduces their polyunsaturation and increases their saturation. But, hydrogenation is a controllable process. One can hydrogenate a lot or a little. Thus, a vegetable oil, 50% of which consisted of the polyunsaturated fatty acid, linoleic, may have been hydrogenated in the process of making margarine so that the polyunsaturation has been reduced to 35 to 40%, but the final product is still a good source of linoleic acid when compared with lard at about 9% polyunsaturated and with butter at less than 3% of polyunsaturates.

An additional component of dietary fat which influences the level of blood lipids is dietary cholesterol. The level of consumption of egg yolk, butterfat, and meat fats in the usual American diet provides from 600 to 800 mg. daily of exogenous cholesterol

Figure 22
Photomicrograph of crystals of human ferritin.

with egg yolks alone contributing two thirds of the total. Foods rich in cholesterol are also restricted in planning fat-modified diets.

Water

Because water forms nearly 70% of the body weight of man, it obviously plays an important part in metabolism. Except for fat storage the whole series of chemical actions that are intimately related to the life of a living organism, animal or vegetable, are ultimately referable to changes that take place in solution. It has been shown that the younger the animal, the richer it is in water. It has also been found that the fatter the animal, the smaller the percentage of water.

Water serves as a solvent to help absorb water-soluble nutrients and eliminate water-soluble waste products via the urine. It is indispensable for the control of body temperature via the evaporation of water from the lungs and from the skin.

Water furnishes no calories or vitamins, but it may provide various minerals—calcium and magnesium in the case of hard water and fluoride in the case of waters that have been fluoridated either naturally or by man.

Under normal conditions, 6 or 7 eight-ounce glasses of fluid (water, tea, coffee, etc.) furnish enough water for the metabolic needs of the tissues of adults. The human being can live far longer without food than he can without water.

Minerals

IRON
The average iron content of a healthy adult is only about 4 grams and yet this relatively small quantity is vitally important.[30] Iron deficiency anemia is a common cause of ill health in the United States and in all parts of the world.

About two-thirds of the iron in the body is present in the blood mainly as hemoglobin and approximately 3% is present as myoglobin. The majority of the remainder is storage iron which is found in the liver, spleen, bone marrow and muscle in the form of ferritin or hemosiderin. Additional minute quantities exist in the respiratory enzymes and in iron-binding protein of the plasma.

The main function of iron is its vital role in the transfer of oxygen at various sites in the body. Iron is an essential component of hemoglobin, the pigment in the red blood cells which carries oxygen from the lungs to the tissues. Iron is present as myoglobin in skeletal and heart muscle where it functions by accepting the oxygen from the hemoglobin and also in peroxidase, catalase and the cytochromes.

Iron is not an element which tends to be either used up or destroyed in the properly functioning body. Unlike some minerals it is not required for excretion and only very small amounts appear in the urine and sweat. Minute quantities are lost in desquamated cells from the skin and intestine, in shed hair and nails and in the bile and other body secretions. The body is however, efficiently economical and conservative in the use of iron. Iron which is released when the erythrocytes are old and broken down is taken up and utilized again and again for the manufacture of new red blood cells. This economy with iron is important. In normal circumstances only about 1 milligram of iron is lost to the body daily by excretion into the intestines, in urine, in sweat or through loss of hair or surface epithelial cells.

Because of the preservation of iron, the nutritional needs of healthy males and post-menopausal females are very small. Women of childbearing age must however, make good the iron lost during menstruation and childbirth and meet the additional requirements

30. Beal, V. A., and Meyers, A. J., *Amer. J. Public Health*, 60:666, 1970.

of pregnancy and lactation. Children have relatively high needs because of their rapid growth which not only increases their body size but also their blood volume.

Sources of iron

Iron is present in a variety of foods of both plant and animal origin. In many foods there is a considerable variation in the value of iron content according to the soil and conditions in which the food is raised. Rich food sources for iron include meat, especially liver, egg yolk and pulses such as beans and peas. However, many other common foods such as green leafy vegetables, whole grain and enriched cereals, vegetables and fish are good sources of iron. Milk, both human and cow's, contrary to the notion that it is the "perfect food," is a poor source of iron.

In the United States many prepared foods such as bread, breakfast cereals and certain baby foods are artificially enriched with iron. An average American adult diet consisting of a variety of common foods bought at a grocery store or eaten in a restaurant or institution would normally contain about 15 milligrams of iron per day. Because of the poor absorption of iron this may be a rather marginal amount.

Absorption of iron

Absorption of iron takes place mainly in the upper portion of the small intestine. Most of the iron enters the blood stream directly and not via the lymphatics. The precise mechanism by which this absorption takes place across the mucosal cells is not known. Evidence indicates that absorption is regulated to some extent by physiological demand. The important factors may be iron stores, hypoxia, erythropoietic activity and level of unsaturated iron-binding protein. Thus, persons who are iron-deficient tend to absorb iron more efficiently and in greater quantities than do normal subjects. This phenomenon has been demonstrated with medicinal ferrous sulphate and with food tagged with radioactive Fe^{59}.

There are several other factors which affect iron absorption[31]. For example, phosphates and phytates in food reduce while ascorbic acid increases iron absorption. Malabsorption syndromes and gastrectomy reduce, whereas pyridoxine deficiency, untreated pernicious anemia and chronic pancreatic insufficiency increase the absorption of iron. A recent report suggests that egg yolk, despite its relatively large amount of iron, inhibits the absorption of iron.

The availability of the iron in foodstuffs is very variable. Healthy subjects normally absorb only 5 to 10 per cent of the iron in their foods whereas iron-deficient subjects may absorb twice this amount. Therefore on a diet consisting of 15 milligrams of iron, 0.75 to 1.5 milligrams of iron would be absorbed in a normal subject but as much as 3 milligrams in an iron-deficient subject. Similarly absorption is generally increased during growth and pregnancy, following bleeding and in other conditions where an enhanced demand for iron exists.

Requirements

From the above it is clear that dietary requirements of iron are in the order of ten times the body's physiologic requirements. If a normal man or post-menopausal woman requires 1 milligram of iron daily due to iron losses then the dietary requirements are about 10 milligrams per day. This allows a fair margin of safety as absorption is increased with need.

Menstrual loss of iron has been estimated to average a little under 1 milligram per day taken over the whole year.[32] The recommendation is that females of child bearing age have a dietary intake of 18 milligrams per day.

The average daily iron requirements necessary to develop the fetus and tissues and to expand the maternal blood supply during pregnancy is about 1.5 milligrams. Most of this additional iron is required in the second and third trimesters of pregnancy.

31. Amine, E. K. and Hegsted, D. M., *Jour of Nutrition 101*:927, 1971.
32. Frenchman, R. and Johnston, F. A., *J. Am. Dietet. Assoc. 25*:217, 1949.

Satisfactory studies have not been made regarding iron requirements or rate of iron absorption during lactation. Human breast milk contains about 0.2 milligrams iron per 100 milliliters, so a woman in full lactation might be losing 1 milligram or more of iron per day.

Infants are born with a store of iron which is adequate for the first three months of life. Premature infants may have a reduced iron store at birth and are therefore more liable to develop iron-deficiency anemia. Recommended daily dietary allowances of iron range from 6 milligrams at age 1 month, up to 15 milligrams for those 1 to 3 years old.

Iron deficiency

A glance at the nutritional requirements for iron and the iron content of commonly eaten foods might suggest that iron deficiency should be rare, but such is not the case. Food iron is poorly absorbed. Iron is not readily excreted into the urine or into the gastrointestinal tract, and severe iron deficiency is usually associated with an increased need for iron; expansion of the total body iron during growth, increased needs associated with pregnancy, or with blood loss. Iron deficiency is most common in young children, in women during the child-bearing age, and individuals with a chronic blood loss. Many people may be unaware or unconcerned about chronic blood loss for example; in mild peptic ulcer, bleeding gums, hemorrhoids, menorrhagia, and in the tropics from hookworm infestation or schistosomiasis. Whenever blood is lost, iron is lost, and if not replaced it will eventually lead to iron-deficiency anemia. See anemias, page 27.

Iron excess

Hemosiderosis is a condition in which excessive accumulations of iron have occurred in the human due to a number of causes. These have included frequent blood transfusions, especially for hemolytic anemia (in this condition the erythrocytes are destroyed but their iron is not lost to the body) and from excessive oral or parenteral doses of therapeutic iron or as a result of excessive consumption of iron in food. For example the diet of Bantu natives of South Africa contains quantities of iron often exceeding 100 mg. per day—the result of using iron utensils in their daily cooking and for the preparation of fermented beverages.[33] It is also seen in hemochromatosis, a disease believed to be due to an inborn error of metabolism in which excessive iron is absorbed from the diet. The danger of excessive ingestion of medicinal iron is constantly present, especially as enthusiastic advertising leads the health-conscious layman to believe that iron is a body strengthener and a tonic. This may result in persons believing that the more that is taken the better for his or her health. A large variety of iron containing medicinal preparations are available without prescription. As a result it is common for some persons to be consuming many times the recommended allowances for iron. Accidental poisoning with ferrous sulphate has sometimes been fatal in children.

In iron overload, the plasma iron content is high, the iron binding capacity is depressed and the percent saturation is nearly complete. Iron overload is unknown from iron fortification of foods.

CALCIUM AND PHOSPHORUS

Although calcium and phosphorus are not chemically related they occur together in the body in a ratio that is nearly constant. About 1.5 per cent of the human body is composed of calcium and 1 per cent of phosphorus. These two minerals are mainly in the bones where the calcium combines with phosphorus as various calcium phosphate salts to form a hard substance which gives the body rigidity. However, the skeleton of the body is not the rigid unchanging structure which it appears to be. In fact the bones contain a cellular matrix and calcium is continuously taken up by the bones and given back to the body. The bones also function as a reservoir for these minerals. Appreciable loss or gain in calcium is usually reflected in similar changes in phosphorus content.

33. Bothwell, T. H. and Bradlow, B. A., *Arch. Path.* 70:279, 1960.

Calcium

The body of a healthy adult contains about 1250 grams of calcium, 99 per cent of which is in the bones and teeth. Calcium is present in the blood serum in small but important quantities, usually about 10 mg. in 100 ml. of serum. A substantial reduction in this amount causes the development of tetany while an increase may lead to respiratory or cardiac failure due to impaired muscle function. Approximately 60 per cent of serum calcium is ionized while the remainder is bound to serum proteins. The extra-cellular fluids and soft tissues of an adult contain approximately 10 grams of calcium.

Sources

A great variety of foods such as whole grain cereal products, leafy vegetables, legumes and nuts contain calcium with particularly rich sources being milk and cheese. Sardines and other small fish in which the bones are eaten are other important sources of calcium.

Cow's milk contains 120 mg./100 ml., considerably more than human breast milk (30 mg./100 ml.).

Absorption

Calcium absorption depends on several factors but vitamin D is one of the most important. Thus, even if the intake of calcium is adequate, calcium absorption is reduced and calcium balance may be negative if the subject is deficient in vitamin D.

Certain amino acids, citric acid and lactose enhance calcium absorption. In contrast, phosphates, phytates and oxalates inhibit calcium absorption. It is doubtful, however, if any of these substances are ordinarily important determinants of the calcium requirements of man.

Of considerable importance in calcium metabolism and calcium requirements is the human power of adaptation. The physical basis of adaptation is not proven but its existence is clear.

People eating low calcium diets have been shown to have a more efficient absorption of calcium than those customarily eating diets higher in calcium. Thus as the intake of calcium is lowered the efficiency of the body to absorb and retain calcium increases, while raising calcium intake results in reduced utilization.

Calcium is present in the feces, urine and sweat, that in the feces being primarily dietary calcium which for a number of reasons has not been absorbed. The amount of calcium in the urine varies greatly but usually is that which has been absorbed but not taken up by the skeleton or soft tissues. Considerable quantities of calcium may be lost in sweat in individuals working at high temperatures.

Requirements

A specific statement of man's calcium requirement is not easy to make because of the "adaptation mechanism," the many other factors influencing absorption, and the variability in calcium loss from the body. The recommended allowances (NAS/NRC 1968) are put at 800 mg. calcium daily for adults, a figure well above theoretical estimates of need.

The FAO/WHO Expert Group[34] suggested that a practical allowance for adults would be an intake of 400 to 500 mg. daily.

Additional calcium is needed during pregnancy and lactation. The fetus has its calcium needs and human breast milk contains 30 mg. calcium per 100 ml. During pregnancy and lactation an extra 500 mg. calcium is suggested above the normal adult recommendation. Without this the woman is likely to deplete her own calcium reserves. This extra calcium is readily supplied by an extra pint of milk.

Children are constantly increasing the size of their skeletons and so have especially high calcium requirements. The recommended dietary allowances are put at 700 mg. for infants (which incidentally is higher than the amount which would be obtained from breast milk) and rises to 1400 mg. daily during the pubertal growth spurt and the teen age period.

34. *Calcium Requirements*, World Health Organization Technical Reports Series No. 230, WHO, Geneva, 1961.

Deficiency

Despite the publicity given to the importance of a high calcium intake and the scientific work done on calcium requirements in adult man there is no convincing evidence to show that a deficiency of calcium even at levels of 250 to 300 mg. daily is harmful. Presumably adults achieve balance at the level of intake supplied by their usual diet, largely because of "adaptation."

In females on a habitually low calcium intake, depletion of body calcium resulting from repeated pregnancies and prolonged lactation may play a role in the development of osteomalacia. However, vitamin D deficiency is far more often implicated in this condition.

Even in children the development of rickets is known to be largely independent of calcium intake. There is still no convincing evidence on whether low calcium intakes, so commonly found in developing countries, adversely affect the growth of children.

Osteoporosis is a common disease of aging in the United States and in many other parts of the world. Loss of bone may be an inevitable process of aging and usually starts in middle age. Although high calcium diets are frequently recommended in osteoporosis and in the diets of the elderly there is not good scientific evidence to show that this measure actually increases bone density. There is now evidence to show that a high intake of fluoride benefits calcium retention and lessens osteoporosis.

Excess

Certain populations such as the Masai in East Africa who consume a diet almost exclusively of milk may have intakes of over 2000 mg. calcium per day. This has not been shown to have any deleterious effects.

However, there are conditions in which excessive calcium is found in the serum, urine or soft tissues such as idiopathic hypercalcemia, the "milk alkali syndrome," renal stone formation, hypercalciuria and fluorosis. At the present time there are no epidemio-logic data to prove that high calcium intakes are responsible for these conditions.

IODINE

The body of an average adult contains about 40 mg. of iodine of which about half is present in the thyroid gland. Iodine is essential for the formation of thyroxine and triiodothyronine, the hormones of this gland.

Sources

Iodine is present in rocks and soils but through the ages much has been washed into the sea. Man gets his iodine from food and from water, which vary in amount according to the iodine content of their source. Thus there are waters with a fairly high content of iodine and others with negligible amounts, and the same foodstuff grown in different soils has a different iodine content.

Seafoods on the whole are rich in iodine and dairy products, eggs, and some vegetables may be good sources. Iodized salt is sold in the United States but housewives are frequently unaware as to whether they are buying iodized or non-iodized salt and even institutions such as hospitals and schools are frequently found to be using non-iodized salt, a most unfortunate situation.

The Food and Nutrition Board of our National Research Council has recommended federal legislation making mandatory the iodization of all salt put up for sale for human consumption. However, there is as yet no federal legislation concerning salt, and state laws are not uniform. A suitable iodine level is 0.5 gram of potassium iodide in 1 kilogram of purified salt.

Absorption and utilization

In normal people, iodine is readily absorbed from the intestinal tract and about one third is utilized by the thyroid gland while two thirds is excreted in the urine. Iodine nutriture can be studied by determining the avidity of the thyroid gland to take up radioactive iodine, by measurement of the stable iodine content of the urine, and by determination of the protein-bound iodine. Iodine in the feces comes mainly from the bile.

Requirements

It has been suggested that 1 microgram of iodine per kilogram body weight is an adequate intake in the human. However, growing children and women during pregnancy and lactation have increased needs.

Deficiency

A deficiency of iodine leads to the development of goiter but there are several other causes of goiter besides iodine deficiency. Endemic goiter which is discussed on page 48 occurs where population groups have dietary sources of iodine below normal requirements. Iodine lack is a major public health problem in many parts of the world[35] as well as in the U.S. due to our laxness in using iodized salt.

Iodine deficiency goiter is really a defense mechanism designed to keep thyroid hormones at an optimal level. A decrease in the circulating iodine-containing thyroid hormones triggers a release of thyroid-stimulating hormone (TSH) from the pituitary gland. This eventually causes a thyroid hypertrophy and an increase in the number of thyroid epithelial cells.

Goitrogens in brassica plants such as cabbage have been shown to increase the needs of iodine in certain laboratory animals. As a result iodine intakes which would be adequate under normal circumstances failed to prevent goiter in those animals consuming large quantities of goitrogens. There is little evidence to show that goitrogens in normal diets have been important in the production of goiter in man.

FLUORIDE

In man fluoride deposition is found mainly in the teeth and the skeleton but the total quantity is small. However the presence of traces of this mineral in the teeth helps to protect them against caries and as such,

35. Follis, R. H., J. Trop. Med. Hyg. 12:137, 1964.

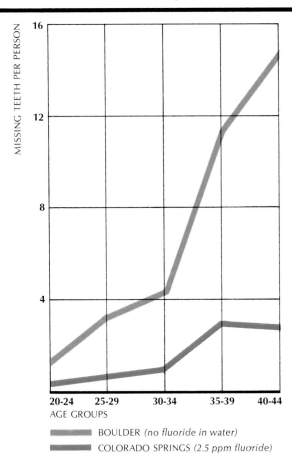

Chart 7
Missing Teeth per Adult
(fluoride and non-fluoride communities)

BOULDER *(no fluoride in water)*
COLORADO SPRINGS *(2.5 ppm fluoride)*

That the benefits of fluoride accrued during childhood are carried over into adulthood is shown by a comparision of missing teeth of adults in Boulder, Colorado (no fluoride in the drinking water) and Colorado Springs (2.5 ppm of fluoride in the drinking water). At age 40-44 the loss of teeth is less than 4 permanent teeth per person in Colorado Springs while it averages about 16 permanent teeth loss per person in Boulder, Colorado. The ratio of tooth loss is 4 to 5 times greater, at all times, in the non-fluoride area than in the fluoride area from age 20 to 44.

Chart 8

Dental Caries and Dental Fluorosis *in relation to fluoride in public water supplies.*

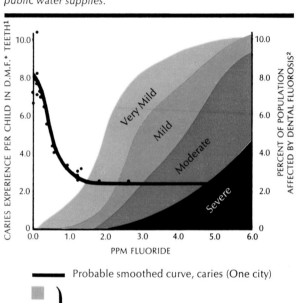

Probable smoothed curve, caries (One city)

} Probable smoothed curves, fluorosis

1. Adapted from Dean, H. T., New York Symposium 1945.
2. Adapted from Dean, H. T., Int. Den. J. 4:311-337, 1954.
*D.M.F. = Decayed, missing and filled.

Figure 23
Moderate fluorosis shown as mottling of the permanent teeth. This 14-year-old drank well water containing 5.5 ppm of fluoride from birth. (5.5 times optimum level)

Figure 24   Skeletal fluorosis. (18 times optimum level)
This resulted from prolonged consumption of water from a stream containing 18 ppm of fluoride. X-ray of forearm shows calcific deposits between the radius and ulna.

fluoride is essential to optimal health and is thus referred to as a mineral nutrient.

The protective effect of fluoride occurs primarily during infancy and early childhood when the teeth are developing but its caries preventive action is carried over into adulthood as long as one has access to fluoridated water. Studies suggest that fluoride has a second role in strengthening bone and that an adequate fluoride intake is important as a protection against osteoporosis.[36]

Recent studies show fluoride is also necessary for growth in rats[36a] and fertility in mice.[36b]

Sources

The main source of fluoride for humans is the water they drink. If this contains around 1 part per million (1 ppm) of fluoride it will supply adequate amounts of this mineral nutrient. Many waters contain quantities of fluoride much less than this and the addition of fluoride (fluoridation) to raise its level in water to what is considered optimal is an important public health measure. Fluoride addition has been shown to reduce the incidence of dental caries by 60 to 70 percent.

Requirements

An intake of about 1-2 milligrams per day is considered adequate. A water supply containing 1 part per million (1 ppm) of fluoride will supply 1 to 2 milligrams per day depending on the consumption of water and other beverages such as coffee, soft drinks, and those reconstituted from frozen citrus drinks.

Deficiency

A deficiency of fluoride during infancy and childhood leaves the teeth relatively unprotected from dental caries. Tooth decay is a major public health problem which has important economic implications.

36. Bernstein, D. S. et al., JAMA 198:499, 1966.
36a. Schwarz, K., Transactions, American Association for the Advancement of Science, 138th Meeting, Dec. 1971.
36b. Messer, H. H., Armstrong, W. D., and Singer, L., Science 177:No. 4052, 893, 1972.

There is increasing evidence of less osteoporosis in areas where the fluoride content of the water is high than in comparable areas where the fluoride content of the water is low. There are good data to show that osteoporosis improves if large doses of fluoride are administered therapeutically. Recent evidence suggests that arterial calcification may be less marked in high fluoride than in low fluoride areas.[37]

Excess

An excessively high intake of fluoride during childhood causes a condition known as dental fluorosis in which the teeth become mottled and somewhat discolored. Very large intakes of fluoride cause bone changes with increased bone density, calcification of muscle insertions and exostoses. This can be diagnosed most easily by radiographic means. The most likely places to find these changes is in x-rays of the *forearm*. (See Figure 24) Dental and skeletal fluorosis do not occur in communities with a properly controlled fluoridated water supply. These conditions are found in certain defined areas of India,[38] Tanzania,[39] the western parts of United States and other areas where the water sometimes contains 10 to 45 ppm of fluoride, well above the level of 1 ppm used in fluoridation. Fluorosis has occasionally occurred in industrial workers as the result of chronic intoxication due to prolonged contact with high concentrations of flouride compounds used in certain manufacturing processes.

SODIUM AND POTASSIUM

Sodium and potassium are essential elements in the human body. Sodium is present in greatest concentration in extracellular fluid. Its role is to maintain equilibrium between the extra and intracellular fluid compartments. Its other functions include its role in maintaining the pH of blood, its involvement with potassium in muscle contractility and the conduction of impulses in nerves. Potassium on the other hand is

37. Bernstein, D. S. et al., ibid.
38. Singh, A. et al., Indian J. Med. Sci. 20:569, 1966.
39. Latham, M. C. and Grech, P., Am. J. Pub. Health 57:651, 1967.

the main cation of the cells and its concentration in the intracellular fluid is greater than in the extracellular.

Sources

Although foods of both animal and plant origin contain sodium the former usually contain more. In U.S. diets most of the sodium usually comes from salt which is added at the table, is cooked with the food or has been added during processing. Thus bacon, ham, sausage, butter and other foods are salted during preparation and foods such as bread have salt added. Man has added salt to his food for over 3000 years but in normal circumstances there appears to be no actual nutritional need for more sodium than is present in raw foods. An increasingly common source of sodium in our diets is monosodium glutamate, which is a flavor enhancer.

Potassium is ubiquitous and is present in most commonly eaten foods. A dietary deficiency of potassium does not occur on an ordinary mixed diet. Bananas, oranges, and some other foods are rich sources of potassium, see Appendix A.

Requirements

The Food and Nutrition Board have not established dietary allowances for sodium or potassium. Intakes of sodium in the U.S. average about 5 grams per person per day, at least 5 times or more above physiological needs (equals about 13 grams of salt).

Intakes of potassium in the U.S. are usually between 0.8 to 1.5 grams per 1000 calories consumed, with minimal needs believed to be between 0.8 and 1.3 grams per day.

Deficiency

Excessive and prolonged sweating from any cause may lead to symptoms and signs of salt depletion if the lost salt is not replaced but only the water. Giddiness, nausea, apathy, exhaustion, cramps (often termed "miner's cramps"), vomiting and finally respiratory failure may result. Such symptoms are prevented when profuse sweating occurs simply by adding a little more salt to food or in extreme cases by adding about 1 gram of salt per liter to the water consumed. Salt tablets are *not* necessary.

Sodium depletion may also result from severe vomiting and diarrhea, during adrenocortical failure, as a result of excessive use of diuretics and in certain renal diseases.

Potassium deficiency is associated with general muscle weakness which may lead to reduced intestinal tone and distention, to cardiac abnormalities, and to respiratory failure. Less severe but chronic depletion results in what is termed "hypokalemic nephropathy." Common causes of potassium depletion are the infectious and nutritional diarrheas[40] of infancy which are often termed "weanling diarrheas." Care must be taken to ensure an adequate potassium intake in those on a restricted diet, those taking diuretics, and hospital patients receiving parenteral nourishment and intravenous fluids.

Excess

There is increasing interest in the role that our unnecessarily high intakes of dietary sodium may play in the etiology of hypertension.

The lethal effects of large intakes of sodium chloride have been reported in several incidents where infants have been accidently fed a saline mixture in place of water, glucose or some other fluid in a formula diet.

MAGNESIUM

Magnesium is an essential constituent of all soft tissue and bone in man. It is an important metallic cation in living cells and is required in enzymes responsible for energy transformation of phosphate bonds. The adult body contains about 25 grams of magnesium, of which approximately 70% is found in the bones. The skeleton appears to provide the body's magnesium stores.

Sources

Most foods, especially those of vegetable origin, contain useful amounts of magnesium. Whole grain

40. Darrow, D. C. *et al.*, *Pediatrics* 3:129, 1949.

cereal products, potatoes, vegetables and fruits provide most of the magnesium in human diets.

Absorption

In contrast to calcium, vitamin D does not aid in magnesium absorption. Failure of absorption is not known to be a problem.

Requirements

The recommended dietary allowance is 300-350 mg. per day for normal adults, 400 mg. per day during pregnancy and lactation and 40-70 mg. per day for infants.[41]

Deficiency

Magnesium deficiency[42] in man has been described. This results in a condition similar to hypocalcemic tetany.[43] Sufferers, usually alcoholics,[44] have low serum magnesium levels and the condition responds dramatically to magnesium administration. Magnesium deficiency has also been described with kwashiorkor.[45]

This deficiency in experimental animals leads to soft tissue calcification and results in increased arterial atherosclerosis in animals on a high cholesterol diet. The role of low intakes of magnesium on atherogenesis in man is unknown. Many U.S. diets are marginal in their content of magnesium.

COPPER

Copper, widely distributed in food, is an essential nutrient required for the formation of hemoglobin as well as the production and survival of erythrocytes. Evidence that ill health due to a dietary deficiency of copper occurs in man is unverified.

In Wilson's disease or hepatolenticular degeneration there is accumulation of excessive copper in the tissues, probably due to a genetic absence of a liver enzyme. It is characterized by neurological degeneration and cirrhotic liver changes. A reduction in dietary copper may be useful in treatment particularly the use of chelating agents to bind free copper.

SULPHUR

Sulphur, an element present in all protein material and, therefore, all living matter in the human, is present mainly in the two sulphur-containing amino acids, methionine and cystine, plus the vitamins thiamine and biotin. Additionally, cells containing sulphate ions and free sulfhydryl (SH) groups are important in some enzyme systems. It is also present in chondroitin sulphate found in cartilage and bone.

It is likely that most of the required sulphur is obtained from dietary methionine and cystine, but some foods, notably onions, are rich in organic sulphur. Little is known of sulphur requirements or sulphur deficiency in man.

TRACE ELEMENTS

It is generally accepted that man has a requirement for zinc, manganese, molybdenum, cobalt, selenium and the elements already discussed. Chromium and bromide may also be required but the evidence is vague.

Much work details the important effects of a deficiency of these elements on experimental animals and there is little doubt that they are also essential to man. Evidence suggests that some effects of deficiency may be found in severe malnutrition, particularly in kawashiorkor where the diet is deficient in protein, calories, and often many other nutrients.

These trace elements are all supplied in adequate quantities in normal diets and chances of deficiency are therefore very slight.

Vegetables (notably green leafy vegetables), cereals, especially if unrefined, liver and kidney, seafood and meat are good sources of most trace elements.

41. *Recommended Dietary Allowances*, 7th Edition, NAS-NRC, Publication 1694, Washington, D.C.,1968.
42. Schroeder, H. A., Nason, A. P., and Tipton, I. H., *J. of Chronic Disease* 21:815, 1969.
43. Vallee, B. E., Wacker, W. E. C., and Ulmer, D. O., *New Eng. J. Med.* 262: 155, 1960.
44. Wacker, W. E. C., Moore, F., Ulmer, D. O., and Vallee, B. E. *JAMA 180:* 161, 1962.
45. Montgomery, R. D., *Lancet* 2:74, 1960.

Vitamins

Vitamins are organic substances—not carbohydrate, fat or protein—which are present in minute quantities in foodstuffs and are necessary for metabolism. They are classified together not because they are chemically related or because they have similar physiological functions but more because of the way in which they were discovered and because in very small amounts they are vital factors in the diet and yet they do not fit into the other categories of nutrients.

VITAMIN A

History

Vitamin A is a fat-soluble vitamin. It was discovered about fifty years ago when scientists found that if the only form of fat in the diet of certain laboratory animals was pork lard the animals ceased growing, whereas on an identical diet in which butter replaced the lard the animals grew and thrived. Clearly there was some substance in the butter which was not present in the lard. This substance seemed to be necessary for the health of the animals even though both diets contained adequate quantities of carbohydrates, fats, proteins and minerals. Further animal experiments showed that egg yolk and cod liver oil contained the same vital food factor which was then named vitamin A.

A little later it was established that many vegetable products had the same nutritional properties as the vitamin A which was present in butter and other animal fats. The plants contained a yellow pigment called carotene which is converted to vitamin A in the human body.

Properties

Vitamin A is soluble in fat but insoluble in water. It is an almost colorless substance and is found only in foods of animal origin.

Carotenes are yellow substances which occur widely in plants. The yellow color of the carotenes is masked in some foodstuffs by the green color of chlorophyll which often is present in close association with it. There are several different carotenes which act as provitamins or precursors of vitamin A. The conversion of these substances into vitamin A takes place mainly in the walls of the intestines but also in the liver and kidney.

The liver acts as the main store of vitamin A in the human and most of the vertebrates, hence the high concentration of this vitamin in fish liver oils.

Vitamin A has several known functions in the human body. Vitamin A aldehyde combines with opsin in scotopic vision. The vitamin participates in synthesis of muco-polysaccharides and release of a protease affecting dissolution of the cartilaginous matrix. It also has a role in reproductive processes.

Units

Vitamin A was originally measured in International Units but on the recommendation of the Food and Drug Administration it is now measured in milligrams. The standard is 0.30 micrograms of vitamin A alcohol or 0.60 micrograms of beta-carotene as equal to one International Unit of vitamin A. W.H.O. states that 2 I.U. of beta-carotene are equivalent to 1 I.U. of vitamin A.

Dietary Sources

Vitamin A itself is found only in animal products and the main natural sources are butter, eggs, milk, liver and some fish.

Many plant foods contain carotene. Good sources are dark green leafy vegetables and various pigmented fruits and vegetables such as tomatoes, carrots, sweet potatoes, pumpkin and papaya. Yellow corn is the only commonly eaten cereal that contains carotene. Red palm oil which is produced and eaten in many tropical countries is an extremely rich source.

In the U.S. vitamin A is added to some foods such as margarine and dried milk powder.

Human Requirements

The Food and Nutrition Board's (7th Ed. 1968) Recommended Daily Allowance for adults is 1.5 mg. (5000 I.U.) and is considered to be provided by 1.2 mg. (4000 I.U.) of beta-carotene and 0.3 mg. (1000 units) of pre-formed vitamin A. Allowances of vitamin A for infants and children are somewhat more liberal in terms of recommended allowances in order to provide for growth and to ensure adequate body stores. For the second and third trimester of pregnancy an added daily allowance of 0.3 mg. (1000 I.U.) and for lactation an added daily allowance of 0.9 mg. (3000 I.U.) above that for the normal are recommended.

There are a number of factors which affect absorption of pro-vitamin A from the intestine. Carotene is poorly utilized in persons on a low fat diet while intestinal diseases such as dysentery, celiac disease and sprue limit the absorption of vitamin A and the conversion of carotene. Persons with obstruction of the bile ducts are likely to become deficient in vitamin A as bile salts are essential for the absorption of vitamin A and carotene.

Deficiency

A dietary deficiency of vitamin A may result in the development of xerophthalmia which may then lead to keratomalacia and blindness. This is a serious public health problem in some parts of the world. (See page 37.)

Early signs of vitamin A deficiency are night blindness and the development of dermatological lesions such as follicular hyperkeratosis and crazy pavement skin. Another sign of vitamin A deficiency, though of limited diagnostic value, are Bitot's spots which occur bilaterally in the eyes and are seen as foamy patches on the lateral side of the cornea. (See Figure 8.)

Toxicity

Hypervitaminosis of vitamin A[46] due to excessive intake has occurred with over-medication of a vitamin preparation, in faddists who include extra large doses of the vitamin in their diet, and in other circumstances where excessive amounts are taken over long periods of time.

The signs and symptoms include lethargy, malaise, abdominal pain, headaches, excessive sweating, and brittle nails. Carotenoid deposits may cause a yellow dyspigmentation of the soles of the feet, the palms of the hands and the naso-labial folds. Increased intracranial pressure and edema may develop.

THIAMINE (VITAMIN B₁)

History

The tale of Eijkman and his chickens, like the story of Jenner and his cow vaccine is a classic example of how an astute observation in an unlikely place has led to a historical landmark in the advancement of science. Working in Batavia, Java (now Djakarta, Indonesia) this Dutch physician noted that hens fed a diet of leftover rice cooked for human consumption developed a disease like beriberi. When fed either a whole grain rice or rice polishings they recovered. Eijkman[47] believed that there was a toxin present in polished rice that could be neutralized by something in rice polishings and he published his findings in 1897. In 1901 Grijns[48] first postulated that beriberi might be due to something lacking in polished rice. In 1916 McCollum and Kennedy[49] reported the finding of a water soluble B vitamin which they believed to be the anti-beriberi factor. This vitamin was subsequently divided into its anti-beriberi and anti-pellagra factors. Finally vitamin B_1, subsequently to be called thiamine, was isolated and then synthesized.

Properties

Thiamine hydrochloride is a compound consisting of a pyrimidine ring joined by a methylene bridge to a thiazole nucleus. The bond between the two rings is weak, with the result that the compound is easily destroyed in an alkaline medium. Thiamine is highly

46. Hillman, R. W., *Am. J. Clin. Nutr.* 4:603, 1956.

47. Eijkman, *Virchow's Archiv 148*:523, 149:187, 1897.
48. Grijns, *Tidjsch. V. Nederl. Indie 41*:3, 1901.
49. McCollum, E. V., and Kennedy, C., *J. Biol. Chem.* 24:491, 1916.

Beribe1ri heart.

Figure 25a
This patient was a chronic alcoholic whose diet had been poor for a long time; polyneuritis and congestive heart failure accompanied cardiac dilation. Thiamine deficiency leads to impaired function and enlargement of the heart, particularly of the right auricle and ventricle, shown by X-ray.

Figure 25b
After 1 week of thiamine therapy.

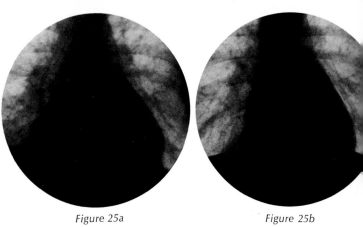

Figure 25a   *Figure 25b*

soluble in water and will resist temperatures up to 100° C. but tends to be destroyed if heated above this. This has practical implications, the vitamin being destroyed in food that is fried in a hot pan or cooked too long under pressure. Because of its solubility, thiamine is easily leached out of food-stuffs being washed or boiled.

Thiamine pyrophosphate functions in carbohydrate metabolism as a coenzyme in the decarboxylation of alpha-keto acids and in transketolase. Without cocarboxylase, pyruvic acid accumulates in various tissues, an occurrence which tends to happen in thiamine deficiency. A specific relationship between thiamine nutrition and transketolase activity at the enzyme or cellular level has likewise been observed in man.[50]

Thiamine is easily absorbed from the intestinal tract but the body is unable to store any quantity of thiamine. The liver, heart and brain have a higher concentration than muscle tissue or other organs. A person on a high thiamine intake soon becomes saturated and begins to excrete increased quantities in the urine.

Units
The activity of thiamine hydrochloride is expressed in milligrams of the chemically pure synthesized substance.

Dietary Sources
Thiamine is found in foods of both animal and vegetable origin. The richest sources among commonly eaten foods are pork, whole grain and enriched cereal grains, and the seeds of legumes. Green vegetables, fish, meat, fruit and milk all contain useful quantities.

In cereals the thiamine is present mainly in the germ and in the outer coat of the seed and much of the vitamin is lost if cereals are milled and refined.

Human Requirements
The recommended daily allowance for thiamine is 0.4 mg. per 1000 calories for all ages with an added allowance of 0.2 mg. daily during the second and third trimester of pregnancy and 0.4 mg. daily during lactation. When the daily calorie intake is less than 2000, an amount of 1.0 mg. is recommended for older adults.

Deficiency
A deficiency of thiamine is the cause of the disease beriberi. This occurs mainly among rice eating peoples and is common in Asia. In the U.S. thiamine deficiency is fairly common in alcoholics and may lead to Wernicke's disease and Korsokoff's syndrome. (See page 38.)

Toxicity
This vitamin when taken in excessive amounts is excreted in the urine and hence has no known toxicity. The kidney has no known threshold.

RIBOFLAVIN
History
Early work on the properties of vitamins in yeast and other foodstuffs showed that the antineuritic factors were destroyed by heat but that a growth promoting factor was not destroyed. This heat stable vitamin was finally isolated from milk and the yellow crystals were named riboflavin. In 1935 it was synthesized by the German chemist, Kuhn, who had also been responsible for its isolation.

Properties
Riboflavin functions as a coenzyme or active prosthetic group of flavoproteins concerned with tissue oxidation and respiration. The vitamin plays an important role in both protein and energy metabolism. Riboflavin is a water-soluble yellow crystalline substance. It is heat stable in an acid solution but decomposes in an alkaline solution or on exposure to sunlight.

50. Brin. M., *Am. J. Clin. Nutr.* 12:107, 1963.

Figure 25c
After 3 weeks' treatment, progressive reduction in heart size is visible.

Figure 25c

In experimental animals a deficiency causes a failure of growth as well as lesions of the skin and eyes.

Units

Riboflavin is measured in milligrams of the chemically pure substance.

Dietary Sources

Many foods of animal and vegetable origin contain riboflavin. The richest sources are milk and its non-fat products. Other good sources are green vegetables, meat (especially liver), fish and eggs. A proportion of the riboflavin is lost when food is cooked, when exposed to sunlight, or if the water in which the food is cooked is discarded. Milk in bottles exposed to direct sunlight loses some of its riboflavin content.

Human Requirements

Recommended daily dietary allowances for riboflavin in the U.S. are set at 1.7 mg. for men and 1.5 mg. for women. An additional 0.3 mg. is recommended for women during the last two-thirds of pregnancy and an additional 0.5 mg. during lactation. Children have relatively higher needs than adults and 0.6 mg. is the recommended allowance during infancy and this ranges up to 1.5 mg. for adolescent boys.

These allowances provide what is considered a reasonable margin of safety. The minimum requirement to prevent clinical signs of deficiency is believed to be about 0.3 mg. per 1000 calories in adults.

Deficiency

Naturally occurring riboflavin deficiency alone has not been shown to cause serious life threatening disease in man. Ariboflavinosis does however lead to lesions of the lips, mouth, eyes, skin and genitalia.[51]

The most common lesions are angular stomatitis and cheilosis of the lips. Angular stomatitis consists of fissures or cracks radiating from the angles of the mouth onto the skin. Sometimes the lesions extend onto the mucous membrane inside the mouth. These cracks have a raw appearance but may become yel-

51. Rivlin, R. S., *New Eng. J. Med. 283*:463, 1970.

Figure 26a
Generalized dermatitis and growth failure in riboflavin-deficient rat. There is marked keratitis of the cornea.

Figure 26b
After one month of treatment with riboflavin the animal shows improvement. Growth has been resumed and ocular and skin lesions are practically gone.

Figure 26c
After two months of treatment the rat shows no signs of the original deficiency.

Figure 27a
Riboflavin deficiency manifested as fissures at angle of mouth.

Figure 27b
Complete eradication after treatment with riboflavin therapy.

lowish due to secondary infection. Cheilosis of the lip is a condition in which there are painful cracks on the upper and lower lips. The lips may be swollen and denuded at the line of closure. The lesions may be red and sore, or dry and healing.

Less commonly, glossitis develops and causes a patchy denudation, papillary atrophy and so-called magenta tongue. These latter conditions are not exclusively due to riboflavin deficiency.

In males scrotal dermatitis (vulval dermatitis in females) has been particularly well described in experimental riboflavin deficiency. The affected skin is usually intensely itchy and tends to desquamate. The resulting scratching leads to redness, excoriation and sometimes infection.

Eye lesions, again not specific to riboflavin deficiency, include vascularization of the cornea, photophobia and lacrimation. The condition may cause an annoying irritation of the eyes with a sensation of itching and burning.

Dyssebacea which is most commonly seen in the naso-labial folds but may involve the nose, the canthi of the eyes and occasionally the ears is a feature of riboflavin deficiency and other conditions. If visualized with a magnifying glass the condition is seen as plugs of yellowish colored keratin standing out from the ducts of enlarged sebaceous glands.

Toxicity

Excess intake of riboflavin spills into the urine. Toxicity in man has not been described.

Figure 28

Figure 29

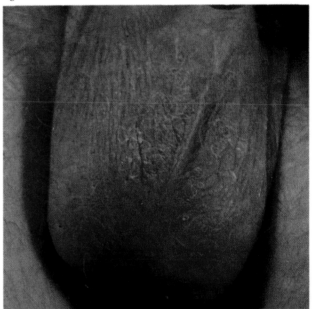

Induced riboflavin deficiency. Twelve of 15 male patients maintained for 9-17 months on a riboflavin-deficient but otherwise adequate diet (0.55 mg. riboflavin daily per 2,200 calories) displayed clinical signs of deficiency including angular stomatitis, seborrheic dermatitis and scaly scrotal skin lesions. Three of the four controls who were on the vitamin-deficient diet supplemented with 2 mg. riboflavin daily, developed scrotal erythema with little or no scaling.

Figure 28

Angular stomatitis with bilateral fissures. Left oral lesion began after about 4½ months on the deficient diet and continued in a fluctuating state of exacerbation and remission for several months. Right lesion appeared 6 weeks after one at left with no preceding infection, and healed in about three weeks without recurrence.

Figure 29

One patient developed scaly pruritic dermatitis on an erythematous base involving only the anterior aspect of the scrotum bilaterally. Other developments in this patient were patchy seborrhea of the scalp, resistant to treatment and vertical fissures around the nostrils following a respiratory infection and progressed to a weeping, crusty lesion. With 6 mg. of riboflavin added to the diet, improvement of the scrotal lesion was prompt and unequivocal; healing of the more chronic lesions was slower but also definite.

Figure 30

Beginning vascularization of the cornea. Vessels of the limbic plexus have proliferated and invaded the cornea. Vascularization may be accompanied by itching, burning, a feeling of grittiness in the eyes, and photophobia. All symptoms and signs regress after treatment with the vitamin riboflavin.

Figure 31
Skin lesions in pellagra.

NIACIN (NICOTINIC ACID)
History

Just as the history of thiamine is linked with the disease beriberi so the history of niacin is inextricably woven with the story of the disease pellagra. The association of beriberi is with the Far East and a rice diet, that of pellagra with the New World and with corn (maize) eating peoples.

Well over 200 years ago Casal attributed pellagra to a poor diet and yet it was not until this century that the nutrient responsible was described and isolated. Confusion was caused in part because the disease pellagra could be cured by a protein rich diet and therefore was thought to be due to a protein deficiency. Later a liver extract almost devoid of protein was shown to cure pellagra and in 1926 Goldberger demonstrated that yeast extract contained a pellagra-preventing non-protein substance. In 1937 niacinamide (nicotinc acid amide) was isolated by Elvehjem and this was found to cure "black tongue," a pellagra-like disease which occurred in dogs.

Properties

Niacin functions in the body as a component of two coenzymes important in glycolysis and tissue respiration. It is a simple derivative of pyridine and is extremely stable. Niacin is a water soluble white compound which is moderately resistant to heat and to both acid and alkaline solutions. It is related chemically to nicotine but has very different physiological properties and is essentially non-toxic. It has recently been found that niacin (but not niacinamide) in very large oral doses will lower serum cholesterol (beta-lipoproteins and triglycerides) in man.

Niacin has been accepted in the United States as the name for nicotinic acid, and niacinamide for nicotinic acid amide.

Units

Niacin is measured in milligrams of the synthesized pure substance.

Dietary sources

Niacin is present in many foods of vegetable origin and niacinamide in most foods from animal sources. Particularly rich are lean meat (especially liver), peanuts, yeast and cereal bran or germ. Like other B vitamins the main source in the diet is frequently the cereal staple consumed. Whole grain or lightly milled cereals contain more niacin than refined cereal grains and flours. Niacin is now often added to many manufactured food products especially those made from cereals.

Beans, peas and other legumes are good sources but starchy roots such as potatoes and cassava (manioc, yucca), common vegetables and fruits and milk are all poor sources of the vitamin.

The human body has the ability to convert the amino acid tryptophan to niacin. It is believed that about 60 mg. of dietary tryptophan is equivalent to 1 mg. of niacin. Diets in the U.S. often contain 600 mg. or more of tryptophan and this provides a substantial contribution to the niacin pool. However, diets of poor persons in the U.S. and elsewhere are usually low in protein and in these people pellagra is likely to occur. The tryptophan content of their diets is often as low as 150 mg.

Corn is poor in niacin and its principal protein, zein, is very low in tryptophan content. There is evidence that some of the niacin in corn is present in a bound form and may be unavailable.

Human Requirements

Because niacin is obtained pre-formed or from tryptophan the recommended allowances are stated as niacin equivalents. These include the pre-formed vitamin and the precursor tryptophan (60 mg. tryptophan representing 1 mg. niacin). Allowances for adults in the U.S. are set at 18 mg. for males and 13 mg. for females with a recommendation of an extra 2 mg. during the second and third trimesters of pregnancy and an extra 7 mg. during lactation. Children have proportionately higher requirements and an intake of 5 to 8 mg. is recommended for infants and up to 20 mg. for adolescent boys.

The recommended allowance based on a calorie intake and expressed in niacin equivalents is 6.6 mg. per 1000 calories and not less than 13 mg. if the daily caloric intake is between 1000-2000.

It is believed that the minimum requirement to prevent pellagra averages 4.4 mg./1000 calories per day or a minimum intake in adults of 9.0 mg. per day particularly if the caloric value is less than 2000 calories.

Deficiency

A deficiency of the vitamin leads to the disease pellagra.

Toxicity

Both niacin and niacinamide may be regarded as non-toxic because there is very wide margin between their therapeutic and toxic doses.

Niacin (but not niacinamide) acts as a vasodilator and therefore may cause a flushing of the skin, dizziness and nausea. These symptoms are temporary and in no way harmful. Because of these vasomotor symptoms, niacinamide is preferable to niacin, especially when large doses are needed for the treatment of pellagra. But as previously mentioned, large doses of niacin lower blood cholesterol where niacinamide does not have this effect.

Figure 32a
Pellagrous dermatitis in advanced stage.

Figure 32b
Same patient after intensive niacin therapy.

Figure 33
Nicotinamide deficiency–advanced pellagra.
Dermatitis of elbows is precipitated by friction and shows initial desquamation in the center of the lesion. With periods of remission, residual pigmentation persists and becomes deeper with repeated attacks.

VITAMIN B_6

Vitamin B_6 is a useful term because it covers three pyridine derivatives all of which occur in food and which are interconverted metabolically in the human. These substances are pyridoxal and pyridoxamine present mainly in animal products and pyridoxine, present mainly in plants.

Properties

Vitamin B_6 is involved in the metabolism of amino acids and it is an essential part of the enzyme glycogen phosphorylase.

Units

The activity of pyridoxine is expressed in milligrams of the synthesized pure substance.

Sources

Vitamin B_6 is widely distributed in foods of both animal and vegetable origin. Whole grain cereals, milk, meat (especially liver and kidney) and certain vegetables are good sources of the vitamin which is easily absorbed.

Requirements

A recommended daily dietary allowance was first set for this vitamin in 1968. The recommended allow- ance for adults is 2 milligrams daily plus an additional 0.5 milligram daily during pregnancy and lactation.

Deficiency

Vitamin B_6 deficiency tends to increase the oxalate excretion in the urine. A vitamin deficiency involving vesical stone formation[52] may occur in certain areas of the world where these are common, e.g., Thailand. Some success in treating renal calcium oxalate calculi with magnesium oxide and vitamin B_6 has been reported.

Vitamin B_6 deficiency in infants manifests itself by hyperirritability, convulsions and anemia. An inborn error of metabolism leading to a dependency on a high intake of vitamin B_6 has been described. It is seen during the first seven days of life and leads to convulsions. Unless treated early with vitamin B_6 the child may become mentally retarded. Vitamin B_6 responsive anemias have been reported in adults.

Increasingly important in clinical medicine is the B_6 deficiency which follows treatment of tuberculosis with isonicotinic and acid hydrazide (isoniazid or INH).[53] This drug apparently leads to increased requirements for vitamin B_6 by interfering with certain activities of pyridoxal phosphate. Patients on a poor diet taking INH may develop a severe polyneuritis which may be both painful and disabling. Administration of pyridoxine in daily doses of 10-20 mg. per day may be useful in preventing this complication of tuberculosis treatment.

There is some evidence that pregnant women develop a deficiency and that vitamin B_6 supplementation may be of value in treating the nausea of pregnancy.

Adequacy of vitamin B_6 nutriture is often assessed by measuring the urinary excretion of tryptophan metabolites, particularly xanthurenic acid following a tryptophan load test.

52. Gershoff, S. N. et al., *Am. J. Clin. Nutr.* 8:812, 1960.
53. Biehl, J. P. and Vilter, R. W., *JAMA 156*:549, 1954.

Figure 34
Oxalate bladder stones in Thailand.

Treatment of convulsions in pyridoxine-deficient infant.

Figure 34
Oxalate bladder stones in Thailand.

Figure 35a
Electroencephalogram of infant during convulsions produced by pyridoxine deficiency.

Figure 35b
Five minutes after pyridoxine administration; color improved and the infant slept.

Experimentally induced B_6 deficiency leads to loss of appetite and weight, general weakness and lassitude and certain symptoms and signs normally ascribed to deficiences of other B vitamins. These include cheilosis, glossitis, peripheral neuritis and skin changes reminiscent of pellagra.

Toxicity

Toxicity to vitamin B_6 has been described in men receiving 300 mg./day, a dose far in excess of any therapy recommended for drug treatment and a dose impossible to receive from foods.

PANTOTHENIC ACID

Properties

Pantothenic acid is a part of coenzyme A and is involved in the release of energy from carbohydrate. It is vital to the synthesis and degradation of sterols, fatty acids and steroid hormones. Pantothenic acid is also involved in the acetylation of choline.

Units

The activity of pantothenic acid is expressed in milligrams of the synthesized pure substance.

Dietary Sources

Pantothenic acid is widely distributed and freely available in ordinary foods so that a deficiency is rare in humans receiving a natural or even a marginally adequate diet.

Deficiency

Various studies on volunteers on a diet deficient in pantothenic acid and with a pantothenic acid antagonist, omega methyl pantothenic acid, develop tiredness, abdominal pain and cramps, nausea, sometimes flatulence and vomiting and paresthesia of the hands and feet.[54]

The "burning feet" syndrome accompanied by severe parathesia and great tenderness of the feet in prisoners-of-war on very poor diets in World War II was believed to be in part due to pantothenic acid deficiency.

Human Requirements

Probably 10 mg. of pantothenic acid daily will satisfy human requirements. Most diets in the U.S. contain around 15 mg. per day, even low cost diets.

Toxicity

Toxicity is not known to occur in man.

Figure 36a
Dermatitis in a chick whose diet was deficient in pantothenic acid. The eyelids, corners of the mouth, and adjacent skin are involved. Feathering is retarded and rough.

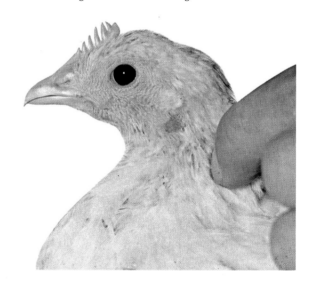

Figure 36b
Three weeks after calcium pantothenate was added to the diet, skin lesions were cured.

54. Hodges, R. E. *et al., J. Clin. Invest. 38*:1421, 1959.

CYANOCOBALAMIN (B$_{12}$)

History

The disease pernicious anemia, so named because it was invariably fatal, was described in detail by Addison in England in 1849. About 40 years ago it was found by Minot and Murphy that the disease improved if the patient consumed raw liver. Soon after this Castle showed that beef mixed with normal gastric juice caused remission in subjects with pernicious anemia but that neither component alone was effective. Castle called the factor in the meat "extrinsic factor." He suggested that the two together interact to produce a substance present in raw liver which relieves pernicious anemia.

It was not until 1948 that the anti-PA vitamin of liver extract was finally isolated independently in England and in the U.S.A. Within a very short time cyanocobalamin (vitamin B$_{12}$) was shown to improve the hematological picture of pernicious anemia as well as to prevent the neurological complication of subacute degeneration of the spinal cord.

Properties

Cyanocobalamin (vitamin B$_{12}$) is a red crystalline cobalt-containing substance which is soluble in water and is resistent to heat. It is readily destroyed by strong acids and alkalis, and also by sunlight. Cyanocobalamin consists of a heavy complex non-protein molecule. In food it is bound to protein and it is now believed that the intrinsic factor, an enzyme secreted by the stomach, removes the B$_{12}$ from its protein combination. It is then absorbed from the small intestine and is stored in the liver and to a lesser extent in the kidney.

Cyanocobalamin is essential for the function of all cells but particularly for cells of the bone marrow, the intestinal tract and the central nervous system. Being active in very small amounts it is an extremely potent catalyst and appears to facilitate reduction reactions such as the conversion of ribose to deoxyribose and of formyl through methyl reduction to tetrahydrofolic

Bone marrow smears in pernicious anemia before and after vitamin B$_{12}$ therapy.

Figure 37a
Smear showing a number of megaloblasts, characteristic of certain anemias.

Figure 37b
Within 48-72 hours after treatment with 25 micrograms of vitamin B$_{12}$ the megaloblasts have been replaced by normoblasts.

acid.[55] It also acts as a cofactor in the transfer of a methyl group to homocysteine to form methionine. It is probably involved in the metabolism of protein, carbohydrate and fat but it is of greatest importance in nucleic acid and folic acid metabolic processes.

Units

Activity of cyanocobalamin is expressed in milligrams and micrograms of the pure crystalline substance.

Dietary Sources

Cyanocobalamin is obtained in human diets from foods of animal origin, particularly meat (liver and kidney are very rich) and dairy products. Negligible quantities are present in foods of vegetable origin. Herbivores obtain their cyanocobalamin from bacterial synthesis in the rumen, but in man intestinal microbial synthesis provides very little of the vitamin.

Cyanocobalamin occurring in food is poorly absorbed in the absence of intrinsic factor. Storage of vitamin B_{12} in the human is good.

Human Requirements

In normal adults a diet containing 5 micrograms of cyanocobalamin daily will satisfy requirements. Diets in the U.S. show marked variation in their content of B_{12}. This is because meat, fish and other animal products are relatively expensive and as a result there are wide class differences in the quantities consumed. High cost diets contain about 31 micrograms and low cost diets as little as 2.7 micrograms of vitamin B_{12}. Absorption is inversely related to the intake of the vitamin in a range from 30 to 70 percent.

Persons with pernicious anemia or with megaloblastic anemia due to dietary lack of cyanocobalamin often respond to as little as 0.1 microgram of the vitamin given by injection.[56] Normally 0.5-2.0 micrograms given daily parenterally will maintain complete remission, but doses of 2-4 micrograms are needed to replenish liver stores. Once saturation has occurred about 1.5 micrograms of cyanocobalamin daily will maintain and satisfy the biochemical needs of the body. Recommended daily dietary allowances are 5 micrograms for adults, 6 micrograms for the elderly, and 8 micrograms during pregnancy.

Deficiency

Pernicious anemia is a manifestation of vitamin B_{12} deficiency but is not due to a straight forward dietary deficiency of the vitamin. There is a defect, probably genetic, which results in impaired secretion of intrinsic factor by the stomach. A constant finding in pernicious anemia is absence or reduced amounts of both intrinsic factor and free HCl in the gastric juice. Pernicious anemia leads to weakness, to oral manifestations and to signs of central nervous system involvement. A soreness of the tongue is often intermittent but when present the tongue is red and inflamed looking and between attacks there is evidence of papillary atrophy. The tongue eventually becomes smooth and glazed. Concomitant with the glossitis are lesions of other mucous surfaces of the mouth including the lips. The neurologic manifestations are indicative of lesions in both the lateral and posterior spinal cord with peripheral nerve degeneration. Pallor, palpitations and eventually more severe cardiovascular disturbances are all features of the anemia.

Gastrectomy if fairly radical may cause a similar condition because the secreting cells of the stomach are removed.

Persons who live exclusively on vegetable products and who do not even eat dairy products and eggs are called vegans or "strict" vegetarians. Most vegetarians commonly consume milk and its by-products and also eggs and are really "lacto-ovo-vegetarians." Vegans are likely to develop most of the signs of pernicious anemia including glossitis and evidence of involvement of the long tracts of the spinal cord but do not usually develop anemia.[57]

55. Silber, R., and Moldow, C. F., *Am. J. Medicine* 48:549, 1970.
56. Castle, W. B., *J. Amer. Med. Assn.* 48:541, 1970.
57. Wokes, F., Badenock, J., and Sinclair, H. M., *Am. J. Clin. Nutr.* 3:375, 1955.

Figure 38
The tongue in pernicious anemia is typically pale and shiny, the papillae having atrophied in the course of the glossitis which is often the first symptom of the disease. The tongue may become red and sore; these symptoms usually subside promptly with therapy, but may recur in a relapse. Adequate therapy restores the tongue's normal color and may partially restore the papillae.

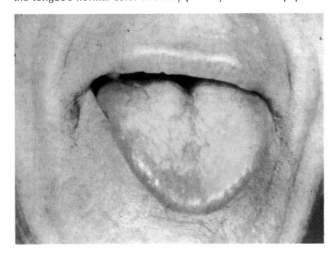

Diphyllobothrium latum, the fish tapeworm, has a propensity for removing cyanocobalamin from the food in the intestine of its host. This may result in megaloblastic anemia which can be cured by injection of the vitamin.

Cyanocobalamin deficiency complicated by a deficiency of folic acid and other nutrients is a feature of sprue and other malabsorption syndromes.

Toxicity

Cyanocobalamin is not toxic to man when given by mouth or injection in amounts very much larger than those recommended for therapeutic purposes.

FOLACIN (Folic acid, folate and pteroylglutamic acid)
History
In the early 1930's, Dr. Lucy Wills, in India, clearly indicated the public health importance of megaloblastic anemia in pregnant women. She also demonstrated good clinical response to some antianemic principle in autolysed yeast. This principle was ineffective in Addisonian pernicious anemia and was different from cyanocobalamin present in liver extract. In 1941 Mitchell and his colleagues in the U.S.

obtained from spinach leaves a substance they called folic acid which was important in the growth of certain microorganisms. A few years later folic acid was synthesized and shown to have a beneficial hemopoietic effect in pernicious anemia. The immediate high hopes were lessened when it was found that folic acid did not prevent the neurological lesions of this disease.

Properties

Folic acid is a yellow substance which is slightly soluble in water. The function of folacin coenzymes is the transfer of single carbon units in intracellular synthesis, particularly of purine and serine.[58,59,60] Folacin is stored mainly in the liver. Blood, serum and urine contain folacin in many different forms and these act as growth factors for certain non-pathogenic bacteria normally present in the human thus complicating physiologic studies of the vitamin.

There has been much research on the precise role of folacin in hemopoiesis. Most evidence suggests that folate deficiency anemia is extremely difficult to produce in mammals unless a folic acid antagonist is administered or certain conditions exist concurrent with the folate deficiency. These include ascorbic acid deficiency, a bacteria-free intestinal tract or a high level of methionine added to the diet.

Units

Folacin activity is reported as milligrams and micrograms of the crystalline pure substance.

Dietary Sources

Dark green edible leaves, kidney, liver, and vegetables are the richest sources of the vitamin in human diets. Smaller amounts are present in meat, cereals, fruits and some roots. Milk, eggs and poultry are poor sources. Storage of food and particularly cooking cause considerable vitamin loss. The vitamin is readily absorbed from the normal intestine.

58. Luhby, A. L. *et al., Advances Metab. Dis.* 1:263, 1964.
59. Herbert, V., *Am. J. Clin. Nutr.* 20:562, 1967.
60. Vilter, R. W. *et al., Am. J. Clin. Nutr.* 12:130, 1963.

Human Requirements

Recommended daily dietary allowances were first set by the Food and Nutrition Board in 1968. The recommendation is 0.4 milligrams of folacin for adults with an additional 0.1 milligram during lactation and an additional 0.4 milligram during pregnancy.

Deficiency

Macrocytic anemia is the main manifestation of folic acid deficiency in the human. It is characterized by lesions of the alimentary tract including stomatitis, glossitis, changes in the intestines, diarrhea and malabsorption.

Megaloblastic anemia of pregnancy occurs because of the increased needs for the vitamin during pregnancy, vomiting which is sometimes persistent during pregnancy, the dietary lack of the vitamin in the diets of some pregnant women and possibly because of a metabolic defect in the production of the folic acid coenzymes.

In sprue and other malabsorption syndromes there is a folate deficiency because of impaired absorption and often megaloblastic anemia is present. This may also be accompanied by vitamin B_{12} deficiency.

A nutritional macrocytic anemia may occur in subjects on an exceedingly poor diet. Megaloblastic anemia may result from a combination of folic acid and vitamin C deficiency in persons with scurvy. Infants on a diet purely of milk may also develop a nutritional macrocytic anemia, as milk is deficient in both folic acid and ascorbic acid.

Megaloblastic anemia in alcoholics may be due to their generally poor dietary habits and is usually associated with low folate intakes. It has been suggested that iron deficiency may also result in a functional defect in folate utilization.

Herbert in 1962 reported on experimental folate deficiency, placing himself on a low folate diet. In four months he developed megaloblastic anemia and other signs of folacin deficiency.[61]

61. Herbert, V., *Tr. Assoc. Am. Phys.* 75:307, 1962.

Perhaps no other nutrient has caused so much debate or confusion as has folacin in causing a dietary deficiency disease in man. It is not absolutely clear whether the deficiency causes or is caused by morphological changes in the intestinal tract. The answer is probably that folacin deficiency induced by some extraneous cause is a more important public health problem than is a true dietary folacin deficiency.

Toxicity

Folacin is not toxic to the normal human even in doses much larger than those usually consumed or even those used as a therapeutic measure. The dangers of doses above 0.1 mg. per day is that they may mask the neurologic manifestations of pernicious anemia. In the United States at the present time it is illegal to sell without a prescription vitamin preparations recommending doses of more than 0.1 mg. folic acid daily.[62] Physicians prescribing folic acid should be aware of this potential danger.

VITAMIN C (ASCORBIC ACID)
History

The history of vitamin C is linked with that of scurvy. This disease was known long before the vitamin era as several centuries ago the anti-scorbutic effects of certain foods were described. In those early days scurvy was a particular scourge of sailors taking voyages of many weeks without fresh food. It was however not until 1747 that James Lind of Scotland demonstrated that scurvy could be cured or prevented by the consumption of citrus fruit. This led, well before the discovery of vitamins, to the inclusion of certain fresh foods and fruits in sailors' diets.

In the 19th century, scurvy began to occur for the first time among infants when they were being fed with the newly introduced powdered and canned

62. *Recommended Dietary Allowances*, 7th Edition, NAS-NRC, Publication 1694, Washington, D.C.,1968.

Megaloblastic anemia of pregnancy treated with folic acid. Patient, 32, hospitalized with severe anemia two weeks after delivery of her fifth child, responded within 48 hours to intravenous folic acid therapy.

Chart 9

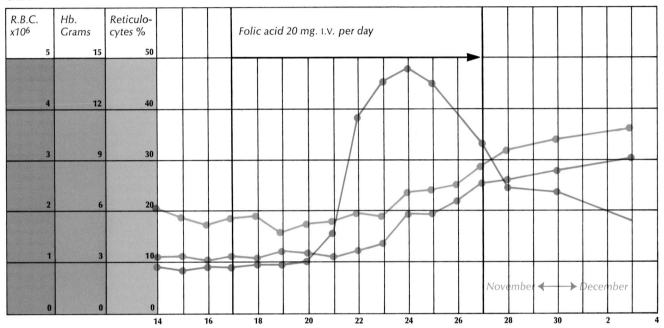

R.B.C. x10⁶	Hb. Grams	Reticulo- cytes %
5	15	50
4	12	40
3	9	30
2	6	20
1	3	10
0	0	0

Folic acid 20 mg. I.V. per day

November ←→ December

14   16   18   20   22   24   26   28   30   2   4

Figure 39a
Inset of peripheral blood illustrates the characteristic poikilocytosis and anisocytosis of untreated macrocytic anemia.

Figure 39b
Illustrates the recovery of the red cells' normal size and shape after therapy. Polymorphonuclear leukocytes, included in the photographs to indicate comparative cell size, also show, prior to treatment, the hypersegmentation typical of macrocytic anemias.

milks instead of the usual diet of breast milk or fresh cows' milk. The vitamin C had been destroyed when these milk products were heated during preparation.

In spite of the value attributed to vitamin C, ascorbic acid wasn't isolated until 1928 and was finally synthesized in 1932.

Properties

Ascorbic acid is a white crystalline substance very highly soluble in water and readily oxidized. It is not affected by light but is destroyed by excessive heat especially in an alkaline solution.

Vitamin C has many functions in the body. The Recommended Dietary Allowances[63] of the Food and Nutrition Board summarizes ascorbic acid's role in the following metabolic systems:

    a) oxidation of phenylalanine and tyrosine via para-hydroxyphenylpyruvate;

    b) hydroxylation of aromatic compounds;

    c) conversion of folacin to folinic acid;

    d) regulation of the respiratory cycle in mitochondria and microsomes;

    e) hydrolysis of alkyl monothioglycosides;

    f) development of odontoblasts and other specialized cells including collagen and cartilage and

    g) maintaining the mechanical strength of blood vessels particularly the venules.

It is the failure of this latter function which leads to several of the signs and symptoms of scurvy including hemorrhage into various tissues.

Units

Ascorbic acid is measured in milligrams and grams. In some textbooks it is still referred to in terms of International Units. The original I.U. was defined as the amount of vitamin C present in 0.1 ml. of lemon juice.

Dietary Sources

Vitamin C is less widely present in foodstuffs than are the other important water-soluble vitamins. In

63. *Recommended Dietary Allowances,* 7th Edition, NAS-NRC, Publication 1694, Washington, D.C.,1968.

Figure 40
Gingival lesions in advanced scurvy.

normal United States diets the main source is from citrus fruits, juices, tomatoes and other fruits and vegetables. Eggs, meat and fish are rather poor sources, as is milk after pasteurization. Dried cereal grains and the seeds of legumes are devoid of vitamin C unless sprouting. Vitamin C is often added to many beverages and some foods and if so, the label will so indicate.

Human Requirements

The daily dietary allowances recommended by the Food and Nutrition Board are 60 mg. for adult males and 55 mg. for females with an additional 5 mg. daily during lactation and pregnancy. Recommended allowances during childhood range from 35 mg. during infancy to 55 mg. during adolescence.

These recommendations almost certainly provide a wide margin of safety and in our opinion ascorbic acid intakes of about two-thirds of the recommended allowances are more than adequate. It should be noted that in Britain the recommended allowance for vitamin C in adults is 20 mg., and in Canada, Australia, and Norway it is 30 mg.

The difference of opinion is because of two schools of thought. Those favoring the higher recommendations believe in saturating the body with the vitamin and those favoring the smaller allowance suggest the amount should be based on that required to maintain good health. There is no evidence that scurvy or poor healing of wounds or any other abnormality occurs on intakes of 20 mg. daily under conditions where there is no increased utilization or decreased absorption of this vitamin.

Deficiency

A deficiency of vitamin C leads to the disease scurvy. (See page 43.) There is some evidence that a subclinical deficiency of the vitamin, not sufficient to cause any of the signs of scurvy, may result in slow healing of wounds or ulcers. Therefore persons undergoing surgery, or following trauma or with persistent ulcers, who are suspected of having a low intake of vitamin C, should have a vitamin C-rich-diet or receive supplemental ascorbic acid tablets.

Claims have been made for the efficacy of large doses of ascorbic acid in preventing the common cold. Controlled trials have shown that the vitamin has no benefit in this regard.

Toxicity

Very high doses of ascorbic acid can be taken without the development of any toxic effects. After saturation is reached the body merely excretes the vitamin in the urine.

VITAMIN D

History

It had been postulated that rickets was a nutritional deficiency disease and for many years prior to any knowledge of the vitamin, cod-liver oil had been successfully used in its treatment. It was not until 1919 that a British scientist, Sir Edward Mellanby, using puppies, demonstrated conclusively that the disease was of nutritional origin and that it responded to a vitamin present in cod-liver oil. This led to some confusion because it was already known that cod-liver oil contained vitamin A. In 1922 McCollum isolated a second fat-soluble vitamin from cod-liver oil and called it vitamin D. Around the same time work had

Figure 41
In scorbutic rosary, the enlarged costochondral junctions of scurvy resemble those of rickets. The lesions in scurvy may feel sharper and may be somewhat tender.

Impaired wound healing.

The first satisfactory controlled experiment in human scurvy was conducted when J.H. Crandon placed himself on an ascorbic acid free diet, supplemented by all other known vitamins, for six months. After three months on the diet, when the ascorbic acid level in the blood had been zero for 44 days, a wound was made in the midback region.

Figure 42a
Biopsy 10 days after this wound shows healing that clinically and pathologically appeared normal, but comparison with Fig. 42c indicates that it was probably suboptimal.

Figure 42b
After six months of the scorbutic diet another wound was made. Biopsy 10 days after second wound shows no healing except of the epithelium (gap in tissues was filled with a blood clot).

Figure 42c
After 10 days of ascorbic acid treatment another biopsy of the second wound shows healing with abundant collagen formation –considerably more than occurred in the first wound.

been proceeding which led to an explanation of how ultraviolet rays prevented rickets.

Properties

A number of compounds, all sterols, possess anti-rachitic properties. Certain sterols which do not possess anti-rachitic properties become anti-rachitic when exposed to ultraviolet light. The two important activated sterols are vitamin D_2 (activated ergocalciferol) which is derived from plants and vitamin D_3 (activated cholecalciferol) which is found in animal tissues.

In human beings when the skin is exposed to sunlight, a sterol compound (7-dehydrocholesterol) is activated to form vitamin D_3 which then becomes available to the body. This activity is identical to vitamin D ingested in the diet. The latter is only absorbed from the gut in the presence of bile.

Vitamin D promotes the absorption of calcium from the gut and is essential to the maintenance of calcium and phosphorus homeostasis, and to the formation of sound teeth and bones.

Units

Vitamin D is measured in International Units. One I.U. is equivalent to the activity of 0.025 μg. of crystalline vitamin D_2 (ergocalciferol) or 0.025 μg. of pure vitamin D_3 (cholecalciferol).

Dietary Sources

Vitamin D occurs naturally only in the fat of certain food products of animal origin. Eggs, cheese, milk, and butter are fairly good sources. Meat and fish contribute small quantities. Fish liver oils are very rich in vitamin D (and vitamin A) but the amounts vary. In the U.S. milk is frequently fortified with vitamin D and many other food products, especially those frequently eaten by children, have vitamin D added. The fortification of these basic foods is a very desirable public health procedure.

Human Requirements

The U.S. recommended daily dietary allowance is 10 μg. (400 I.U.) of vitamin D during childhood and in women who are pregnant or lactating. No allowance is set for normal adults but it is presumably of the same order or even somewhat less.

The requirement of vitamin D in adults is not really known. Probably the amounts needed are so low that the requirement can be easily met by the average diet and by casual exposure to sunlight. Vitamin D requirements have been studied most extensively in infants and it is now believed that 7 μg. to 10 μg. (300 to 400 I.U.) daily permits maximum retention of calcium. Premature infants are more prone to develop rickets than are full-term infants and their vitamin D intake should be watched. Adults, particularly aging adults, should receive an average of 400 I.U. daily to assist in absorption of calcium and in maintaining the calcification of their bones.

Adequate intakes of vitamin D are particularly important throughout the growth period and the recommended allowance of 10 μg. (400 I.U.) daily provides a comfortable margin of safety.

Any generalized statement about dietary requirements of vitamin D is difficult because of the variable contribution of vitamin D obtained from exposures of the skin to sunlight. Therefore persons who because of their mode of life or dress receive little skin irradiation from sunlight have higher dietary needs for this vitamin. This applies to persons working at night, to nuns whose clothing covers most of their skin and to individuals from certain cultures such as sects of Muslim where women are often heavily veiled and where they, and often their young children, remain confined indoors or in dark courtyards.

Deficiency

A deficiency during childhood leads to rickets or later in adult life to osteomalacia.

Toxicity

Because supplementary vitamin D is added to many foods in the U.S. and elsewhere, intakes well above the recommended dietary allowances for vitamin D are common. Therefore, when vitamin D prep-

Figure 43
Early skeletal deformities of rickets can persist throughout life. Bowlegs that curve laterally indicate that the weakened bones have bent after the second year, as the result of standing. If severe rickets occurs before the child walks, it produces a combination of bowed thighs and knock-knees.

Figure 44
The rachitic rosary is, next to craniotabes, the earliest sign of rickets. Enlargement of the costochondral junctions results in beads or knobs that can sometimes be seen and can always be felt or demonstrated by X-ray, as in Figure 45 (another infant).

Figure 45
X-ray of infant with rachitic rosary, showing enlargement of the costochondral junctions.

arations are also provided medicinally the total intake may become very high.

The fat-soluble vitamins, unlike the water-soluble vitamins, are not excreted or metabolized and intakes greater than required tend to accumulate in the body.

Excessive quantities of vitamin D, of the order of 2000 I.U. or more per kilogram body weight per day can be toxic to adults or children and may lead to hypercalcemia and its attendant complications.[64] Although some infants with hypercalcemia may be hypersensitive to vitamin D or may have an inborn error of cholesterol metabolism, many undoubtedly show a true intoxication with vitamin D. There is little rationale in exceeding the recommended dose of 400 I.U. or 10 μg./day during infancy.

In children an early common symptom of excessive vitamin D is anorexia and vomiting. The child though refusing food is very thirsty and there may be polyuria. Weight loss and irritability are common and the condition may eventually lead to death. In vitamin D toxicity the level of ionized calcium in the blood is raised. Because of this increased calcium blood level, abnormal calcification may occur in soft tissues, primarily in the walls of blood vessels but also in the kidneys, lungs and other organs.

VITAMIN E
Properties
The metabolic role of vitamin E is not fully understood but it appears that the vitamin functions as an antioxidant at the tissue level. The term vitamin E is used to mean any mixture of physiologically active tocopherols.

Dietary Sources
Vitamin E is found widely in foods eaten by man. The richest sources are vegetable oils. Vitamin E is also present in fresh greens and many other vegetables.

64. Report of the Committee of Nutrition, American Academy of Pediatrics, *Pediatrics* 31:512, 1963.

Human Requirements

In the absence of definite information about human needs for vitamin E as an antioxidant, it is difficult to make a definitive recommendation of vitamin E requirements. They are believed however, to vary between 10 and 30 mg. per day for adults. The breast-fed child receives about 0.5 mg. of vitamin E per kilogram body weight and this has been suggested as the minimum requirement for infants. Vitamin E requirements are increased by the consumption of polyunsaturated fats, but these fats are also good sources of the vitamin.

Deficiency

Experimentally in the rat, vitamin E deficiency often results in sterility. The female rat conceives normally but the fetuses die during gestation and are reabsorbed. The sterility is reversible with vitamin E therapy. In male rats a deficiency of vitamin E leads to a permanent degeneration of testicular germinal epithelium. No similar findings have ever been described in man.

In man, creatinuria noted in patients with cystic fibrosis and xanthomatous biliary cirrhosis has been reduced by administration of alpha-tocopherols. A marked reticulocyte response simultaneous with a decrease in creatinuria has been reported in a small series of Jordanian children suffering from protein-calorie malnutrition who were treated with vitamin E.

Experimental deficiency of vitamin E in man leads to a decrease in the levels of tocopherols in the blood and excessive hemolysis occurs in red blood cells that are treated with hydrogen peroxide in vitro. The clinical significance of this, if any, is not known.

The common belief among laymen that vitamin E is "the sex vitamin" and will reduce sterility and increase potency in man, or that it is useful in the prevention and treatment of heart disease, is not based on scientific fact. It is one of the falsities of nutrition information which is given wide publicity mainly by the numerous food quacks and charlatans. There is

Resorption of fetus in the female rat—vitamin E deficiency.

Figure 46a
Normal rat with well-developed fetuses, 16 days pregnant.

Figure 46b
Vitamin E deficient rat at the 16th day; uterine enlargements represent remains of autolyzed fetuses and placentae.

no good evidence that vitamin E has any value in lessening muscular fatigue or in the treatment of any kind of heart disease.

Reference Standard

One milligram of dl-alpha-tocoperol acetate is equal to one International Unit of vitamin E according to the National Formulary, 1965. There is no U.S.P. standard for vitamin E.

Toxicity

Little is known about the effects of an excessive intake of tocopherol in man, but there is no evidence of toxicity.

VITAMIN K

Properties

Vitamin K is a fat-soluble vitamin which is necessary for the maintenance of prothrombin, a key substance in blood clotting. The molecular action of vitamin K remains an enigma but apparently it acts in the liver in the synthesis of proteins concerned with clotting. The vitamin is believed to be active in stimulating oxidative phosphorylation in tissues, possibly between DPNH and a cytochrome in electron transport.

Dietary Sources

Vitamin K is ubiquitous in human foods though in very small amounts. Most vitamin K is absorbed after being synthesized by human bacterial flora. Dietary deficiency in man rarely occurs.

Human requirements

The Food and Nutrition Board has not established a daily allowance for vitamin K. It is believed that the microgram amounts obtained from the intestinal flora and from good food are sufficient to maintain a normal prothrombin concentration. The exception to this is newborn infants who have vitamin K deficiency in the first few days of life because their intestinal flora is not yet well established and because the mother had been lacking in adequate supplies of the vitamin.

65. *Recommended Dietary Allowances,* 7th Edition, NAS-NRC, Publication 1694, Washington, D.C.,1968.

Deficiency

Although there has been considerable debate it is now generally believed that vitamin K administration to newborn infants decreases the incidence of neonatal hemorrhage. This is especially true in premature infants or newborns with anoxia.[65] A single parenteral dose of 1-2 mg. of vitamin K or one of its analogues is recommended immediately after delivery.[66] Infants born to mothers on anti-coagulant therapy should receive 2-5 mg. vitamin K or its analogue.[67]

The most serious complication of vitamin K deficiency in infancy is cerebral hemorrhage. Some suggest that the incidence could be greatly reduced by

Figure 47
Hemorrhagic disease of the newborn, resulting from vitamin K deficiency in the first few days of life; death in this case was caused by subdural hemorrhage.

66. Moore, C. V., in *Modern Nutrition in Health and Disease,* edited by Wohl and Goodhart, 1968.
67. Ibid.

the routine administration of vitamin K to women during the last two months of pregnancy.

Because vitamin K is fat-soluble any defect in intestinal absorption of fats may lead to vitamin K deficiency. Bile salts are necessary for the absorption and an obstruction of the common bile duct may lead to a deficiency. This has resulted in severe bleeding following surgical intervention to relieve the obstruction. In this situation vitamin K should be given prior to the surgery.

In various malabsorption syndromes (sprue, celiac disease, pancreatic fibrosis and idiopathic steatorrhea) there is poor absorption of fat and therefore of vitamin K. A similar though less severe deficiency can result from ulcerative colitis, regional ileitis and surgical operations in which much of the intestinal tract is excised.

Toxicity

Excessive doses of synthetic vitamin K have led to hemolytic anemia and kernicterus in the infant and for this reason a dose above 5 mg. of vitamin K should not be given to the newborn. As 1 mg. is usually adequate, there is no reason to use such large doses.

BIOTIN

Biotin is essential in many enzyme systems in animals and man. Biotin deficiency does not occur in man except under very abnormal circumstances.

The vitamin is present in many foods and is synthesized in sufficient quantity by human intestinal bacteria to satisfy normal requirements. Daily needs are probably 150-300 micrograms, an amount provided by most diets.

Raw egg white contains a substance called avidin which when combined with biotin makes it unavailable to the body. Biotin prevents "egg white injury" which is a biotin deficiency that can be produced in animals fed a diet high in egg white. Spontaneous biotin deficiency is an extremely rare condition occurring occasionally in an individual who for some strange reason has consumed a diet consisting mainly of raw eggs. It has also been reported in infants whose intestinal tract has been cleared of biotin synthesizing bacteria by injudicious use of sulfa drugs or antibiotics. The presenting sign of biotin deficiency is an exfoliative dermatitis which responds to biotin.

Experimental biotin deficiency in volunteers led to fatigue, depression, malaise, anorexia, muscle pain, nausea, signs of neuropathy and an erythematous scaling dermatitis. These symptoms and signs disappeared when biotin was administered.

Unit Standard

The activity of biotin is expressed in micrograms of the chemically pure substance.

Toxicity

Exceedingly large doses of biotin given to animals do not produce any toxicity. As chemical biotin deficiency is unlikely and no therapeutic dose is recommended, biotin toxicity appears very unlikely.

Egg white injury is a biotin deficiency produced by feeding a rat egg white, which contains a biotin antagonist, avidin.

Figure 48a
The resulting dermatitis, which begins around the eyes and produces the characteristic "spectacle eye," has progressed in the rat to generalized alopecia.

Figure 48b
The same rat three weeks after adequate amounts of biotin were added to the diet. Growth has resumed and skin lesions are improved.

Figure 48c
After three months of treatment, the animal is normal.

Addendum to Second Printing

It is pleasant to note the favorable acceptance this manual has received from students of medicine, health, and dentistry, as well as from allied health workers and the general public. But we wish to emphasize, this is not a textbook on nutrition. It is a brief manual which hopefully will arouse interest to learn more about nutrition, a frequently neglected yet important area of medicine and health.

In this second printing we have corrected a few printing errors, (one picture was "upside down" but few noticed it) and we added sections, one on contemporary food faddism and one on lactose intolerance.

Food Faddism

Faddism, quackery, and charlatanism in food and nutrition have been around a long time and no doubt will continue to be. Basically this is because everyone thinks he is an authority on food because all of us eat. We all have had various personal experiences (both good and bad) with food and we want to share these experiences with others. Some want to share them for a fee and with a little exaggeration. But this is not scientific nutrition, it is testimonial, hearsay, fantasy and (for a few) a lucrative business.

Dictionaries define a fad as a silly thing followed with an exaggerated zeal. A quack is a pretender to skill, particularly in health and medicine, and a charlatan is a quack who is also a vendor of remedies.

Faddism, quackery, and charlatanism exist all over the world from the witch doctors of darkest Africa to plush suites on Park Avenue. They are characterized by countless numbers of bizarre diets to lose weight, by the use of many colored pills for reducing (some combinations of which are really dangerous), by tonics and nutritional supplements to increase appetite and "build one up". Food faddism is particularly rife among trainers and athletic coaches, from high school through professional teams.

Vitamin C, vitamin E, and food referred to as natural, organic, health, macrobiotic, and Dr. So and So's quick weight loss diets are all trying for top place on the totem pole of nutritional nonsense. We all need vitamin C,—30 to 60 mg. daily and we easily get this amount from a balanced diet with a little citrus fruit or tomatoes. But, doses of 500, 1,000, or 10,000 mg. daily are pure quackery. These huge amounts will not effect one's susceptibility to the common cold and they may carry potential harm. We all need vitamin E in amounts varying from 10 to 30 I.U. daily and we easily get this amount from a varied diet. Amounts of 100, 500, or 1,000 I.U. per day will not prevent or treat any kind of heart disease, sexual impotence, muscle cramps, or anything else.

So-called "natural, organic, and health foods" currently are having quite a re-birth in food quackery. All foods are natural or made from natural foods but this is not the same as saying that all nutrients are natural. For example, vitamin C is natural as it is found in citrus fruits and is synthetic when added to many non-citrus juices or drinks but in both cases it is identical in chemical composition and physiologic action. As Gertrude Stein would have said, vitamin C is vitamin C, is vitamin C. So-called imitation meats are usually made from textured soybean protein and hence are also made out of a natural food.

All foods are "organic" in that they are made of organic compounds; carbon, hydrogen, and oxygen. All food are "health foods" in that as part of a balanced diet they contribute to health.

But, what the devotee (or promotor) of natural, organic, or health foods has in mind are foods grown with the aid of manures and composts, not chemical fertilizers; foods grown without the use of chemical pesticides; and foods not processed with the aid of chemical additives such as preservatives, anti-oxidants, and various flavoring and coloring agents. Some people believe that such foods are more healthful but there is not a shred of evidence to support their beliefs or the testimonials they are so eager to give. There is increasing concern that much of food quackery is filled with chicanery and fraud. This in part is because the profits are high.

Macrobiotic means "large or long life" but the original macrobiotic diets based largely on brown rice and severe restriction of fluid cause just the opposite. There is in the medical literature, documented evidence of severe ill health and death from following such nutritional nonsense to the extreme. Macrobiotic diets are usually combined with a certain amount of pseudo-oriental philosophy which seems to give the diets a scientific aura they do not deserve. The so-called macrobiotic diets which drastically restrict fluid and are limited to very few foods are *dangerous* and should not be followed by anyone for any length of time.

While macrobiotic diets have only taken their place in food faddism in recent times, the Mayo Diet has been around for at least a generation. Let us emphasize that this diet is usually referred to as the Mayo Diet, *not* the Mayo Clinic Diet. It did not originate with the Mayo Clinic and has been a constant source of embarrassment to that well respected clinic.

What is the Mayo Diet? "Eggs, bacon, and grapefruit, all you can eat, but nothing else, and we guarantee you will lose weight. The grapefruit has peculiar and special properties that help burn up fat, including stored body fat, so that calories are lost". What nutritional nonsense! Grapefruit is a good citrus fruit but it is no big yellow spark plug metabolizing fat. Personally we think the Mayo Diet dangerous because of the large amount of saturated fat and cholesterol.

The many "quick weight loss diets", even though some are promoted by physicians have no scientific validity. True, one will lose weight because of the sheer boredom of eating the very limited choice of foods or because of the nauseating effect of the usually high fat content of the diets. These diets do not train one in proper eating habits. They offer too much saturated fat. They do not provide good nutrition. They do not stress the equally important part of more physical activity (exercise) in achieving weight loss. Weight is promptly gained when one goes off these "odd ball" diets. They are another example of contemporary quackery and charlatanism.

Lactose Intolerance

Lactose is the sugar in milk, a disaccharide, and lactase is the intestinal enzyme necessary for its metabolism. If the quantity of lactase is low (or absent) lactose cannot be metabolized and thus absorbed. It slowly passes through the bowel where the normal bacterial flora ferment it to organic acids, thus changing the pH of the stool, gas is formed, an osmolar flow of water is directed into the intestine and one has considerable abdominal distress, often accompanied by diarrhea.

An intolerance to lactose should not be confused with gastrointestinal milk allergy. This latter condition results from a sensitivity to milk, and usually to the milk protein beta-lactoglobulin. The disease manifests itself in early infancy and the prevalence is low, probably less than 1 percent.

In contrast, lactose intolerance is more prevalent and is mainly seen later in childhood or even adulthood. In nearly all humans, lactase activity is high in infancy. However, in the non-white races, as in most other mammals, lactase activity often drops to low levels following weaning and remains low through adulthood. A majority of Caucasians, and possibly some other races, who continue to drink milk beyond infancy, have high levels of the enzyme throughout life.

Lactase deficiency, which is more correctly termed low lactase activity, is of three types:

1. *Congenital lactase deficiency*. This is a rare clinical condition in which diarrhea develops soon after birth.[68] The failure to utilize lactose leads to malnutrition and wasting. If diarrhea persists, and it is accompanied by vomiting, there is a loss of fluid and electrolytes. When the milk is withdrawn, and is replaced by a lactose-free diet, the diarrhea disappears, and the infant begins to thrive.

2. *Secondary low lactase activity*. A reduced level of intestinal lactase activity is often found secondary to other disease states, in which there is damage to the microvilli of the brush border of the intestinal mucosa.[69] Many gastrointestinal diseases prevalent in tropical and non-tropical countries affect intestinal enzyme activity in this manner. In developing countries diarrheal disease and protein-calorie malnutrition are important causes of reduced disaccharidase activity. Elsewhere gastroenteritis, ulcerative colitis, infectious hepatitis, peptic ulcer surgery, neomycin administration and other conditions may also lead to secondary low lactase activity.

3. *Primary low lactase activity*. This is a relatively common condition in non-white populations in the United States and other parts of the world.[70] In people with this condition milk was usually well tolerated in early childhood due presumably to high levels of lactase activity but in later childhood and in adulthood levels of this enzyme are low. This condition cannot be termed an abnormality or disease because it is found in 80 to 90 percent of persons of Asian or African origin, in a majority of other non-white peoples, in 5 to 20 percent of Caucasians, and in practically all mammals including the non-human primates.

Lactase activity is usually assessed either using a lactose load test followed by serial measurements of any rise in blood glucose above the fasting level or by intestinal biopsy and determination of enzyme activity levels in the mucosal specimen.

Symptoms and signs are similar whether the lactose intolerance is congenital, primary or secondary. They include abdominal pain or cramps, diarrhea, and flatulence or bloating. These signs frequently occur in persons with low levels of enzyme activity soon after consumption of 50 grams of lactose, the amount usually given in the fasting state in adult lactose load tests. Some of these subjects may also have similar symptoms when they drink milk.

Although more research needs to be done, evidence suggests that many persons with low lactase activity can consume milk without any problems arising.[71] This may be due to the development, over time, of a tolerance to unabsorbed lactose and the products of its breakdown in the intestinal tract. Whatever the mechanism it seems that *milk is not contraindicated* as a useful dietary supplement in populations where low levels of lactase activity are prevalent. It is advisable, however, to be aware that symptoms of intolerance could arise, to introduce milk in gradually increasing amounts, and to have an alternative protein-rich mixture available for the treatment of cases of protein-calorie malnutrition where diarrhea is aggravated by milk.

68. Holzel, A. Sugar malabsorption due to deficiencies of disaccharidase activities and monosaccharide transport. *Arch. Dis. Child.* 42:341, 1967.

69. Crane, R. K. A perspective of digestive-absorptive function. *Amer. J. Clin. Nutr.* 22:242, 1969.

70. Bayless, T. M. and Christopher, N. L. Disaccharidase deficiency. *Amer. J. Clin. Nutr.* 22:181, 1969.

71. Protein Advisory Group of the United Nations, Milk Intolerance—nutritional implications, Document 1.27/9 1972.

Finale

Now that many of our more serious infectious diseases can be prevented, controlled, and well treated, it is possible that good nutrition is the single most important factor influencing our health.

For example, cardiovascular disease is today the most frequent cause of death and many believe nutrition to be importantly concerned with the prevention and treatment of both atherosclerosis and hypertension, two of the most common diseases in this category. The use of fluoride to prevent dental caries has been one of the great nutritional triumphs of recent years, but still much remains to be done educationally to make this discovery as effective as it should be. Not only are there many children not receiving adequate amounts of fluoride, but iron deficiency anemia, one of the first deficiency diseases to be recognized, is still common in the United States.

In other parts of the world, primarily the underdeveloped areas, lack of total calories, protein-calorie malnutrition of early childhood, a host of infectious diseases made worse by poor nutrition, iodine deficient goiter, anemias due not only to a lack of iron but also to folic acid, and blindness due to lack of vitamin A are examples of major health problems directly concerned with improper or poor nutrition.

It does seem strange that instruction in nutrition is almost nonexistent in most of our medical, dental, public health, and nursing schools. Why? Perhaps because historically, and even today, emphasis has been on getting sick people well, not keeping well people well. The President's Commission on Heart Disease, Stroke, and Cancer recommends bringing better medical care to many areas that do not now have it, obviously most desirable, but not a word about the prevention of these diseases or the improvement of what might now be considered good health.

In the decade before World War II and for a few years thereafter, nutrition was one of the most active fields of research. This was undoubtedly stimulated by medicine's becoming conscious of the great amount of nutritional disease existing in the United States, particularly in the South, but also in the North and by no means confined to the economically distressed. Also, at this time the vitamins, which had been rather mysterious substances in which some medical scientists only half believed, were becoming clearly defined entities with clinically recognizable deficiency syndromes and even their biochemical functions were beginning to become apparent, e.g., Warburg's yellow enzyme, important in cellular respiration, was being related to Vitamin B_2, riboflavin.

In an incredibly short time, the vitamins were purified, their chemical structures defined and means of synthesizing them developed so that they were available in pure form for the treatment and prevention of deficiencies. Through the cooperation of biochemists, clinicians, manufacturers and public health officials, acute vitamin deficiencies declined rapidly and by the end of World War II they were no longer a major cause of morbidity.

Then the science of nutrition suffered a curious fate. It seemed unable to perpetuate itself. There was no one taking the place of Goldberger, Spies, Sydenstricker, Elvehjem and Jolliffe, to mention only a few outstanding workers of the time. Why? Surely one could not conclude that because the field had made spectacular progress, that nothing remained to be done? However, one gains the impression hearing some of the current generation rallying against the need for vitamin supplements that they do not really believe that a serious nutritional problem ever existed or can ever exist again. Surely the idea that the average "homo ineptus" eats an adequate diet simply because it is available, is naiveté unworthy of any scientist. True, the fortification of some of our common foods with various vitamins and minerals–white flour with three B-vitamins and the mineral iron, prepared cereals with various vitamins and minerals, margarines with vitamin A, some milks with vitamin D–has no doubt been important in lessening some nutritional deficiencies. While now only occasionally do obvious nutritional deficiencies force themselves on our attention, there is no satisfactory evidence that in their milder and more subtle forms they may not still be common. Furthermore, what evidence have we that we have obtained the ultimate in salubrity through diet? Further food fortification may be the answer here.

Perhaps it is thought that since the release of energy from food is a biochemical problem, nutrition will be adequately dealt with by the biochemists. True, much of biochemistry has nutritional significance and biochemical research is constantly uncovering facts that bear on nutritional problems. Nevertheless it would seem desirable that someone gather these facts together and apply them to practical clinical problems. After all, in a practical way, we would be badly off without engineers in spite of our competent physicists.

While vitamin deficiencies may no longer be a pressing problem in the United States, there are other nutritional problems which are, such as obesity, deficiency anemias, too much saturated fat and salt, and possibly the whole problem of trace elements as exemplified by the lack of fluoride in our foods and waters. The nutrition surveys currently in progress in various parts of the United States are indicating that 5 to 20% of the population show various signs of mild vitamin and mineral deficiencies so we may have more nutritional deficiencies than we think.

While we control the blood sugar of diabetics with reasonable facility and prevent them from dying of acidosis, we still fail to prevent many of the serious sequelae, and are these perhaps nutritional inadequacies, excesses as well as deficiencies?

And how do we get good instruction into our medical schools so the physician of tomorrow will do a better job than the physician of today? There have been numerous conferences on this in recent years with much verbiage, many generalities and few positive results. The answer is very simple, employ a few qualified people to teach nutrition. Any medical school that receives an endowed professorship of nutrition will soon be teaching it. It is just that simple.

There is much to nutrition that relates directly and indirectly to health, to poor health if nutrition is poor, to good health if nutrition is good. The purpose of this manual is to interest medical students, physicians, and dentists in nutrition, in the important role good nutrition has to play in the health of their patients and themselves; to outline a few of the principles of modern nutrition; but primarily to stimulate all to learn more about nutrition, to practice it themselves and to get their patients and friends to do likewise.

Suggested References

Present Knowledge of Nutrition. Nutrition Foundation, Inc., 1967.
Nutrition: An Integrated Approach. Pike, R. L. and Brown, M. L., John Wiley & Sons, 1967.
The Family Guide to Better Food and Better Health. Deutsch, R., Creative Home Library, 1971.
Modern Nutrition in Health and Disease, 5th Ed. (Goodhart, R. S. and Shils, M. E., Eds.) Lea and Febiger (in press).
Human Nutrition and Dietetics, 5th Ed., Passmore, R., Williams and Wilkins (in press).
U.S. Nutrition Policies in the Seventies (Mayer, J., Ed.), Freeman & Co. (in press).

Appendices

APPENDIX A

TABLE OF SODIUM, POTASSIUM AND MAGNESIUM CONTENT OF SELECTED FOODS[1]

Food	Amount	Gms.	Na mg.	K mg.	Mg mg.
Apple, raw	1 med.	150	2	165	8
Apricot, raw	1 med.	40	Trace	112	5
Avocado, raw, cubed	¼ cup	36	1	217	16
Bacon:					
fried or broiled	2 slices	14	143	33	4
Canadian, fried or broiled	2 ounces	57	1456	246	14
Banana, raw	1 med.	150	2	555	50
Beans, baked (no pork)	1 cup	187	632	501	69
Beef, lean, cooked	4 oz.	113	68	418	33
Bread:					
Rye, regular	1 slice	23	128	33	10
Rye, unsalted	1 slice	23	7	26	10
White, enriched	1 slice	23	117	24	5
White, unsalted	1 slice	23	7	41	5
Whole wheat	1 slice	23	121	63	18
Whole wheat, unsalted	1 slice	23	7	53	18
Butter:					
Regular	1 pat	7	69	2	Trace
Unsalted	1 pat	7	Trace	2	Trace
Cabbage, raw, shredded	1 cup	73	15	170	10
Cantaloupe or honey dew	½ whole, med.	385	46	966	62
Carrots, raw	1 med.	50	24	171	12
Cauliflower, raw	1 cup	104	14	307	25
Celery, raw	1 stalk	40	50	136	9
Cereals:					
Cornflakes	1 cup	28	281	34	5
Puffed rice, unsalted	1 cup	14	Trace	14	—
Puffed wheat, unsalted	1 cup	14	Trace	48	—
Cheese:					
Cheddar	1 ounce	28	196	23	13
Cottage, creamed	1 cup	225	515	191	—
Cherries, sweet or sour	1 cup	130	3	248	10-18
Chicken, cooked:					
White meat	4 ounces	113	72	498	22
Dark meat	4 ounces	113	97	363	—
Chocolate, bitter	1 ounce	28	1	232	82
Chocolate Syrup	1 Tbsp.	20	10	56	13
Coffee, instant dry powder	1 tsp.	1	1	33	5

TABLE OF SODIUM, POTASSIUM AND MAGNESIUM CONTENT OF SELECTED FOODS[1]

Food	Amount	Gms.	Na mg.	K mg.	Mg mg.
Corn, sweet:					
Cooked	1 ear	100	15	165	—
Canned	1 cup	169	399	164	32
Crackers:					
Graham	1 square	7	47	27	4
Soda, 2″ square	2 squares	8	88	10	2
Egg, whole	1 med.	50	61	65	6
Fish:					
Cod, broiled	4 ounces	113	124	460	32
Haddock, fried	4 ounces	113	200	393	27
Halibut, broiled	4 ounces	113	151	593	—
Tuna, water packed	½ cup	115	47	321	—
Grapefruit sections	1 cup	194	2	262	23
Grapes, slip skin	1 cup	153	5	242	20
Honey, strained	1 Tbsp.	21	1	11	1
Ice cream, vanilla	1 scoop	71	45	129	10
Jam, jelly (assorted)	1 Tbsp.	20	3	16	2
Lamb, any cut, broiled or roasted	4 ounces	113	79	328	21
Lettuce, iceberg	1/6 head	43	4	75	5
Lobster, cooked	4 ounces	113	237	203	25
Macaroni, plain, cooked	1 cup	140	1	85	25
Margarine:					
Regular	1 pat	7	69	2	—
Unsalted	1 pat	7	Trace	1	—
Milk:					
Whole, 3.7% fat	1 cup	244	122	351	32
Skim	1 cup	246	123	354	34
Evaporated, unsweetened	1 cup	252	297	764	63
Noodles, cooked	1 cup	160	3	70	—
Olives:					
Green	1 med.	6	144	3	1
Ripe	1 med.	6	45	2	—
Onions, mature, raw	1 slice	17	2	27	2
Orange	1 med.	180	2	360	20
Orange juice	1 cup	249	3	498	27
Pancakes, from mix	1 med.	45	203	70	—
Peaches, raw	1 med.	114	1	230	11

TABLE OF SODIUM. POTASSIUM AND MAGNESIUM CONTENT OF SELECTED FOODS[1]

Food	Amount	Gms.	Na mg.	K mg.	Mg mg.
Peanuts, roasted, unsalted	1 ounce	28	1	196	49
Peanut butter	1 Tbsp.	16	97	104	28
Pears, raw	1 small	75	2	98	5
Peas:					
Canned, regular	1 cup	160	378	154	32
Frozen	1 cup	160	184	216	38
Canned, low sodium	1 cup	160	5	154	38
Pickles:					
Dill	1 med. whole	100	1428	200	12
Sweet	1 small whole	20	105	—	Trace
Pineapple:					
Raw, diced	1 cup	140	1	204	18
Canned, heavy syrup	2 slices	122	1	117	10
Plums, raw	1 med.	60	Trace	102	5
Pork:					
All cuts, lean, cooked	4 ounces	113	74	441	26
Ham, cured, cooked	4 ounces	113	1051	368	19
Sausage, cooked	1 link	20	192	54	3
Potatoes:					
Peeled, boiled, unsalted	1 med.	122	2	348	27
French fried, unsalted	10 pieces	57	3	486	14
Mashed, milk added	1 cup	195	587	509	23
Potato chips	10 med.	20	200*	226	—
Pretzels	1 med.	20	336	26	—
Pumpkin, canned, unsalted	1 cup	228	5	547	27
Raisins, uncooked	1 snack pack	18	5	137	6
Rice:					
Cooked, regular, salted	1 cup	193	722	54	15
Cooked, unsalted	1 cup	193	4	54	15

TABLE OF SODIUM, POTASSIUM AND MAGNESIUM CONTENT OF SELECTED FOODS[1]

Food	Amount	Gms.	Na mg.	K mg.	Mg mg.
Salad dressings:					
French	1 Tbsp.	15	206	12	2
Italian	1 Tbsp.	15	314	2	—
Mayonnaise	1 Tbsp.	15	90	5	Trace
Russian	1 Tbsp.	15	130	24	—
Shrimp, cooked	4 ounces	113	210	259	58
Syrup, Maple	1 Tbsp.	20	2	35	2
Spinach, cooked	1 cup	180	90	583	113
Squash, Summer, cooked, unsalted	1 cup	136	1	192	22
Strawberries, raw	1 cup	144	1	236	17
Sweet potato, baked	1 potato	110	13	330	34
Tangerine, raw	1 med.	114	1	144	—
Tomato, raw	1 med.	120	4	293	17
Tomato juice:					
Canned	1 cup	242	484	549	24
Canned, low sodium	1 cup	242	7	549	24
Tomato Catsup:					
Regular	1 Tbsp.	17	228	63	4
Low sodium	1 Tbsp.	17	1-6	63	4
Turkey, roasted	4 ounces	113	147	415	32
Veal, all cuts, cooked	3 ounces	85	68	425	15
Watermelon, 1/16 med. melon	1—4″ x 8″ wedge	925	9	925	74
Yogurt	1 cup	244	124	349	—

* Varies greatly according to amount of added salt
(—) denotes unknown
(1) Cooper's Nutrition in Health and Disease. J. B. Lippincott Co., Toronto, 1968

TABLE OF NUTRITIVE VALUES OF THE EDIBLE PART OF FOODS[1]

(Dashes show that no basis could be found for computing a value although there was some reason to believe that a measurable amount of the constituent might be present.)

Food, approximate measure, and weight (in grams)	Approx. Measure	Grams	Water %	Calories	Protein* gm.	Fat* (Total lipid) gm.	Fatty Acids* Saturated gm.	Fatty Acids* Unsaturated Oleic gm.	Fatty Acids* Unsaturated Linoleic gm.	Carbo-hydrate* gm.	Calcium mg.	Iron mg.	Vitamin A I.U.	Thiamine mg.	Riboflavin mg.	Niacin mg.	Ascorbic Acid mg.
MILK, CREAM, CHEESE; RELATED PRODUCTS																	
Milk, cow's:																	
Fluid, whole (3.7% fat)	1 cup	244	87	161	9	9	5	2	Trace	12	285	Trace	366	.07	.41	.2	2
Fluid, nonfat (skim)	1 cup	246	90	88	9	Trace	—	—	—	12	295	Trace	Trace	.10	.44	.2	2
Cheese:																	
Cheddar	1 oz. slice	28	37	113	7	9	5	3	Trace	1	213	.3	372	Trace	.13	Trace	0
Cottage creamed	1 cup	225	78	239	31	10	5	2	Trace	7	212	.7	383	.07	.56	.2	0
Ice cream, vanilla	1 scoop	71	62	147	3	9	5	3	Trace	15	87	.1	369	.03	.13	.1	1
EGGS																	
Raw, whole	1 med	50	74	78	6	6	2	3	Trace	Trace	26	1.1	562	.04	.12	Trace	0
MEAT, POULTRY, FISH, SHELLFISH; RELATED PRODUCTS																	
Beef, cooked:																	
Rump Roast: Choice grade																	
Lean and fat	4 oz	113	48	268	18	21	10	10	1	0	8	2.4	39	.05	.14	3.3	0
Lean only	4 oz	113	60	120	17	6	3	3	Trace	0	7	2.2	11	.04	.13	3.0	0
(visible fat removed at table)																	
Sirloin Steak, Choice grade, broiled																	
Lean and fat	4 oz	113	38	382	23	32	16	15	1	0	10	2.8	50	.06	.18	4.6	0
Lean only	4 oz	113	56	135	21	5	2	2	Trace	0	8	2.5	7	.06	.17	4.2	0
(visible fat removed at table)																	
Hamburger, broiled																	
Regular grind	3 oz	85	54	243	21	17	9	8	Trace	0	9	2.7	34	.08	.18	4.6	0
Ground round	3 oz	85	61	226	25	13	6	5	Trace	0	10	3.0	26	.07	.19	4.8	0
Corned beef, med. fat	3 oz	85	44	316	19	26	13	11	1	0	8	2.5	—	.02	.15	1.3	0
Pork, cooked:																	
Ham, baked																	
Lean and fat	4 oz	113	54	250	18	19	8	10	1	0	8	2.2	0	.40	.15	3.1	0
Lean only	4 oz	113	62	135	18	7	3	4	Trace	0	8	2.3	0	.42	.16	3.2	0
(visible fat removed at table)																	
Roast Pork																	

Lamb, cooked:

Food	Measure	g		Calories													
Roast leg, choice grade	4 oz	113	54	206	19	14	8	5	Trace	0	8	1.2	0	.11	.20	4.0	0
Veal, cooked: Cutlet, medium fat	3 oz	85	60	235	28	13	6	5	Trace	0	9	3.6	0	.10	.27	5.4	0
Chicken, cooked: Fryer, ¼ whole, med.		85	54	255	38	10	3	5	1	0	15	2.3	215	.08	.45	12	0
Fish, cooked: Swordfish, broiled	3½ oz	100	65	174	28	6	—	—	—	0	27	1.3	2,050	.04	.05	10.9	0
Tuna, packed in oil	½ cup	115	61	223	33	9	3	2	2	0	9	2.1	91	.05	.13	13	—
Shrimp	4 oz	113	70	132	28	1	—	—	—	Trace	130	3.5	68	.01	.03	2.0	—
Bacon, broiled or fried	2 slices	14	8	96	4	7	2	4	1	Trace	2	.4	0	.08	.04	.8	0
Frankfurter, cooked	1 med	51	58	152	6	14	—	—	—	1	3	.8	—	.08	.10	1.3	—
Liver, calf, broiled	4 oz	113	51	221	33	7	—	—	—	4	15	16.1	37,114	.27	4.73	19	42

VEGETABLES AND VEGETABLE PRODUCTS

Asparagus, cooked	1 cup	181	94	36	4	Trace	—	—	—	7	38	1.1	1,629	.29	.33	2.5	47
Beans: Lima, cooked	1 cup	166	71	164	10	Trace	—	—	—	32	33	2.8	382	.12	.08	1.7	28
Snap, green, cooked	1 cup	125	92	31	2	Trace	—	—	—	7	63	.8	675	.09	.11	.6	15
Baked, with tomato, molasses	1 cup	187	76	309	14	8	2	2	Trace	45	134	4.8	148	.16	.09	1.4	2
Beets, cooked	1 cup	167	91	52	2	Trace	—	—	—	12	23	.8	33	.05	.07	.5	10
Broccoli, cooked	1 cup	164	91	43	5	1	—	—	—	7	144	1.3	4,100	.15	.33	1.3	148
Cabbage: Coleslaw, raw	1 cup	120	83	119	1	9	1	2	5	10	52	.5	180	.06	.06	.4	35
Cooked	1 cup	146	94	29	2	Trace	—	—	—	6	64	.4	190	.06	.06	.4	48
Carrots, cooked, diced	1 cup	160	91	50	1	Trace	—	—	—	11	53	1.0	16,800	.08	.08	.8	10
Cauliflower, cooked	1 cup	125	93	28	3	Trace	—	—	—	5	26	.9	75	.11	.10	.8	69
Celery, raw	1 stalk	40	94	5	Trace	Trace	—	—	—	1	12	.1	72	.01	.01	.1	3
Corn, sweet Cooked	1 ear	100	73	91	3	1	—	—	—	21	3	.6	400	.12	.10	1.4	9
Canned	1 cup	169	81	140	5	2	—	—	—	32	5	1.0	676	.19	.17	2.2	12
Cucumbers, raw, whole	1 small	100	96	15	1	Trace	—	—	—	3	25	1.1	250	.03	.04	.2	11
Lettuce, leaf	1 med	10	94	2	Trace	Trace	—	—	—	1	4	.1	59	.01	.01	.1	1
Mushrooms, canned	1 cup	161	93	31	2	Trace	—	—	—	6	13	1.3	Trace	.03	.39	3.2	—
Onions, cooked	1 cup	197	92	57	2	Trace	—	—	—	13	47	.8	79	.06	.06	.4	14
Parsnips, cooked	1 cup	211	82	139	3	1	—	—	—	31	95	1.3	63	.15	.17	.2	21
Peas, cooked	1 cup	160	82	114	9	1	—	—	—	20	32	3.2	1,002	.45	.15	2.8	22
Peppers, sweet, green	1 shell	62	93	13	1	Trace	—	—	—	3	5	.4	239	.05	.05	.3	73
Potatoes, medium:																	

(Continued on next page)

Food	Measure	Grams	Water (%)	Food energy (cal)	Protein (g)	Fat (g)	Saturated (g)	Oleic (g)	Linoleic (g)	Carbohydrate (g)	Calcium (mg)	Iron (mg)	Vitamin A (IU)	Thiamin (mg)	Riboflavin (mg)	Niacin (mg)	Ascorbic acid (mg)
Baked, peeled	1 potato	99	75	93	3	Trace	—	—	—	21	9	.7	Trace	.10	.04	1.7	20
Peeled, boiled	1 potato	122	83	79	2	Trace	—	—	—	18	7	.6	Trace	.11	.04	1.5	20
French-fried	10 pieces	57	45	156	2	8	2	2	4	21	9	.7	Trace	.07	.05	1.8	12
Mashed with milk and margarine	1 cup	195	80	183	4	8	4	3	Trace	24	47	.8	332	.16	.10	2.0	18
Potato chips	10 med	20	2	114	1	8	2	2	4	10	8	.4	Trace	.04	.01	1.0	3
Pumpkin, canned	1 cup	228	90	75	2	1	—	—	—	18	57	.9	14,590	.07	.11	1.4	11
Radishes	4 small	40	94	7	Trace	Trace	—	—	—	1	12	.4	4	.01	.01	.1	10
Sauerkraut, canned	1 cup	188	93	34	2	Trace	—	—	—	8	68	.9	94	.06	.08	.4	26
Spinach, cooked	1 cup	180	92	46	6	1	—	—	—	7	186	4.4	16,200	.14	.28	1.0	56
Squash, summer, cooked, diced	1 cup	136	96	19	1	Trace	—	—	—	4	34	.5	530	.07	.11	1.1	14
Sweet potatoes, baked	1 potato	110	64	169	3	1	—	—	—	39	48	1.1	9,720	.11	.08	.8	26
Tomatoes, raw	1 med	120	94	25	1	Trace	—	—	—	5	15	.6	1,021	.07	.05	.8	26
Tomato juice, canned	1 cup	242	94	47	2	Trace	—	—	—	11	17	2.2	1,976	.12	.07	2.0	40
Tomato catsup	1 tbsp	17	69	18	Trace	Trace	—	—	—	4	4	.1	238	.02	.01	.3	3
Turnips, cooked, diced	1 cup	196	94	40	1	Trace	—	—	—	9	52	.7	Trace	.05	.09	.8	48
FRUITS AND FRUIT PRODUCTS																	
Apples, raw	1 med	150	85	64	Trace	1	—	—	—	16	8	.3	99	.03	.02	.1	4
Apple juice	1 cup	249	88	116	Trace	Trace	—	—	—	29	15	1.5	—	.02	.05	.2	2
Apricots																	
Raw	1 med	40	85	21	Trace	Trace	—	—	—	5	7	.2	1,134	.01	.02	.3	4
Canned	4 halves; 2 tbsp. syrup	122	77	103	1	Trace	—	—	—	26	17	.5	2,777	.03	.03	.6	6
Avocados, raw, cubed	¼ cup	36	74	59	1	6	1	3	1	4	13	.2	103	.04	.07	.6	5
Bananas, raw	1 med	150	76	88	1	Trace	—	—	—	23	8	.7	196	.05	.06	.7	10
Blackberries, raw	1 cup	144	84	84	2	1	—	—	—	19	46	1.3	288	.04	.06	.6	30
Cantaloupe	½ med	385	91	56	1	Trace	—	—	—	14	26	.8	6,290	.08	.06	1.1	61
Cherries, raw, sweet	1 cup	130	80	108	2	1	—	—	—	27	34	.6	169	.08	.09	.6	15
Cranberry juice	1 cup	250	83	161	Trace	Trace	—	—	—	41	12	.7	Trace	.02	.02	Trace	99
Fruit cocktail, canned	1 cup	229	80	137	1	Trace	—	—	—	36	21	.9	321	.05	.02	1.1	5

PIES

Fruit ... 1/7 of ... 135 ...

Food	Measure	g															
Mince	1/7 cut	135	43	366	3	16	4	10	1	56	38	1.9	Trace	.18	.11	1.2	1
Pumpkin	1/7 cut	130	59	274	5	15	5	7	1	32	66	1.2	3,211	.12	.18	1.3	Trace

FATS AND OILS

Food	Measure	g															
Butter	1 pat	7	16	50	Trace	6	3	2	Trace	Trace	1	0	230	—	—	—	0
Margarine	1 pat	7	16	50	Trace	6	1	3	1	Trace	1	0	230	—	—	—	0
Cooking Fats:																	
Lard	1 Tbsp	14	0	126	0	14	5	6	1	0	0	0	0	0	0	0	0
Vegetable fats	1 Tbsp	13	0	106	0	12	3	8	1	0	0	0	—	0	0	0	0
Salad Dressings:																	
Commercial, mayonnaise																	
type	1 Tbsp	15	41	65	Trace	6	1	1	3	2	2	Trace	33	Trace	Trace	Trace	—
French	1 Tbsp	15	39	72	Trace	7	1	1	3	2	2	Trace	—	—	—	—	—
Mayonnaise	1 Tbsp	15	15	93	Trace	11	2	3	6	Trace	2	.1	36	Trace	.01	Trace	—
Salad or Cooking Oils:																	
Corn	1 Tbsp	14	0	125	0	14	1	4	7	0	0	0	—	0	0	0	0
Cottonseed	1 Tbsp	14	0	125	0	14	4	3	7	0	0	0	—	0	0	0	0
Olive	1 Tbsp	14	0	125	0	14	2	11	1	0	0	0	—	0	0	0	0
Safflower	1 Tbsp	14	0	125	0	14	1	2	10	0	0	0	—	0	0	0	0
Soybean	1 Tbsp	14	0	125	0	14	2	3	7	0	0	0	—	0	0	0	0

SUGARS AND SWEETS

Chocolate, plain	1 oz	28	1	147	2	9	5	4	Trace	16	65	.3	77	.02	.10	.1	Trace
Honey	1 Tbsp	21	17	64	Trace	0	0	0	0	17	1	.1	0	Trace	.01	.1	Trace
Jams, jellies, preserves	1 Tbsp	20	29	55	Trace	Trace	—	—	—	14	4	.3	Trace	Trace	.01	Trace	1
Syrup	1 Tbsp	20	24	58	0	0	0	0	0	15	9	.8	0	0	0	0	0
Sugar	1 Tbsp	12	Trace	46	0	0	0	0	0	12	0	Trace	0	0	0	0	0

MISCELLANEOUS ITEMS

Food	Measure	g															
Beer (3.6% alcohol)	1 bottle	340	92	171	2	0	0	0	0	16	15	0	0	Trace	.11	.8	0
Carbonated beverage	8 oz	240	90	90	0	0	0	0	0	23	—	—	0	0	0	0	0
Nuts:																	
Peanuts, roasted	1 oz	28	2	160	8	13	3	6	4	5	10	.9	—	.07	.04	5.4	0
Peanut butter	1 Tbsp	16	2	87	4	7	1	4	2	3	9	.3	—	.02	.02	2.4	0
Pizza (cheese)	1 (5½" pc)	75	45	184	7	5	2	3	Trace	27	117	.7	303	.05	.13	.8	5
Popcorn with margarine	1 cup	28	3	155	2	12	3	7	2	11	5	.4	462	—	.02	.3	0
Soups, canned:																	
Noodle type	1 cup	250	93	68	4	2	Trace	1	1	8	10	.8	113	.03	.05	1.0	Trace
Tomato	1 cup	245	90	88	2	3	—	—	—	16	15	.7	1,005	.05	.05	1.2	12

(1) Prepared from "Table of Food Values," by Jelia Witschi, M.S., Harvard Nutrition Service, Department of Nutrition, 665 Huntington Avenue, Boston, Mass. 02115
* Values rounded

APPENDIX C

APPROXIMATE CHOLESTEROL CONTENT OF SELECTED FOODS
(Values from National Diet-Heart Study, 1965)

Item	Portion	Size	Cholesterol per Edible Portion
		gm.	**mg.**
Beef, cooked, trimmed	4 oz.	113	102
cooked, untrimmed	4 oz.	113	113
Brains, cooked, no fat added	3 oz.	85	2674
Butter	1 pat	7	20
Cheese: Cheddar and Processed	1 oz.	28	45
Cottage, Creamed	1 cup	225	23
Cream	1 oz.	28	36
Spreads and Cheese Foods	1 oz.	28	39
Chicken, Turkey, cooked	4 oz.	113	85
Cream: Light (20% fat)	1 tbsp.	15	11
Half and Half (12% fat)	1 tbsp.	15	6
Egg: Whole	1 med.	50	235
White	1 med.	33	0
Yolk	1 med.	17	235
Fish, lean and medium fat, cooked	4 oz.	113	79
very fat, cooked	4 oz.	113	90
Gefilte Fish	3 oz.	85	54
Heart, cooked	3 oz.	85	119
Ham, cooked, trimmed	4 oz.	113	102
cooked, untrimmed	4 oz.	113	113
Ice Cream	1 scoop	71	43
Ice Milk	1 scoop	71	4
Kidney, cooked, no fat added	3 oz.	85	298
Lamb, cooked, trimmed	4 oz.	113	102
cooked, untrimmed	4 oz.	113	113
Lard and other animal fat	1 tbsp.	14	14-17
Liver, cooked, no fat added	3 oz.	85	213
Margarine, all vegetable fat	1 pat	7	0
Mayonnaise and mayonnaise-type salad dressing	1 tbsp.	14	8
Milk: Fluid, whole	1 cup	244	27
Fluid, skim	1 cup	246	0
Pork, cooked, trimmed	4 oz.	113	102
cooked, untrimmed	4 oz.	113	113
Shellfish: Clams, Crab, Lobster, Mussels, Shrimp, cooked	4 oz.	113	170
Sweetbreads, cooked	3 oz.	85	249
Tongue, cooked fresh	3 oz.	85	119
cooked smoked	3 oz.	85	179
Veal, cooked, trimmed	4 oz.	113	102
cooked, untrimmed	4 oz.	113	113

Note: Cholesterol is not present in foods of plant origin such as fruits, vegetables, cereal grains, legumes, nuts or oils.

OBESITY STANDARDS FOR CAUCASIAN AMERICANS[1]

(minimum triceps skinfold thickness in millimeters indicating obesity)[2]

Age (years)	Skinfold measurements	
	Males	Females
5	12	14
6	12	15
7	13	16
8	14	17
9	15	18
10	16	20
11	17	21
12	18	22
13	18	23
14	17	23
15	16	24
16	15	25
17	14	26
18	15	27
19	15	27
20	16	28
21	17	28
22	18	28
23	18	28
24	19	28
25	20	29
26	20	29
27	21	29
28	22	29
29	23	29
30-50	23	30

[1] Adapted from Seltzer, C. C., and Mayer, J. A simple criterion of obesity. *Postgrad Med.* 38 : A 101-107, 1965.

[2] Figures represent the logarithmic means of the frequency distributions plus one standard deviation.

TABLE OF DESIRABLE WEIGHTS FOR MEN AND WOMEN AGED 25 AND OVER

(in pounds according to height and frame, in indoor clothing)

	Height		Small Frame	Medium Frame	Large Frame
	Feet	Inches			
MEN	5	2	112-120	118-129	126-141
	5	3	115-123	121-133	129-144
	5	4	118-126	124-136	132-148
	5	5	121-129	127-139	135-152
	5	6	124-133	130-143	138-156
	5	7	128-137	134-147	142-161
	5	8	132-141	138-152	147-166
	5	9	136-145	142-156	151-170
	5	10	140-150	146-160	155-174
	5	11	144-154	150-165	159-179
	6	0	148-158	154-170	164-184
	6	1	152-162	158-175	168-189
	6	2	156-167	162-180	173-194
	6	3	160-171	167-185	178-199
	6	4	164-175	172-190	182-204
WOMEN	4	10	92- 98	96-107	104-119
	4	11	94-101	98-110	106-122
	5	0	96-104	101-113	109-125
	5	1	99-107	104-116	112-128
	5	2	102-110	107-119	115-131
	5	3	105-113	110-122	118-134
	5	4	108-116	113-126	121-138
	5	5	111-119	116-130	125-142
	5	6	114-123	120-135	129-146
	5	7	118-127	124-139	133-150
	5	8	122-131	128-143	137-154
	5	9	126-135	132-147	141-158
	5	10	130-140	136-151	145-163
	5	11	134-144	140-155	149-168
	6	0	138-148	144-159	153-173

Desirable weight tables are based on the concept that once growth in height has ceased there is no biological need to gain weight and that the best health prognosis (as reflected by mortality and morbidity data) is found in individuals of average or less than average weight in their early 20's. Desirable Weight Tables are designed to be applied to individuals aged 25 and over; measurements are with indoor clothing and shoes.

The Chart is adapted from insurance tables which are derived from the 1959 Build and Blood Pressure Study, Society of Actuaries. Three frame sizes are used, with a range of weights for each rather than a single weight. Unfortunately, no indication is given as to how to estimate frame size.

Acknowledgements

David B. Coursin, M.D.
Lancaster, Pennsylvania and
J.A.M.A. 154:406, 1954
Figures 35a, 35b

John H. Crandon, M.D.
Boston, Massachusetts
Figures 42a, 42b, 42c

William J. Darby, M.D.
Nashville, Tennessee
Figure 38

M. Edward Davis, M.D.
University of Chicago
Printzker School of Medicine
Chicago, Illinois
Figure 47

Thomas R. Dawber, M.D.
Boston, Massachusetts and
Ann. N.Y. Acad. Sci. 107:539, 1963
Chart 1a

James M. Dunning, D.D.S.
Boston, Massachusetts and
Harvard University Press
Chart 8

Bernard S. Epstein, M.D.
Long Island Jewish Hospital
New Hyde Park, New York
Figures 14, 18a, 18b, 18c, 45

Stanley N. Gershoff, Ph.D.
School of Public Health,
Department of Nutrition
Harvard University
Boston, Massachusetts
Figures 34, 4c

Sam Granick, Ph.D.
Rockefeller University
New York, New York
Figure 22

M. K. Horwitt, Ph.D.
St. Louis University
School of Medicine
St. Louis, Missouri and
Arch. Int. Med. 87:682, 1951
Figures 28, 29

Normal Jolliffe, M.D. and
The Upjohn Company
Figures 12a, 12b

Michael C. Latham, M.D.
Graduate School of Nutrition,
Cornell University
Ithaca, New York
Figures 1, 3a, 3b, 4, 6, 11
19, 20, 21, 24, 31

Robert F. Littlefield, Jr.
School of Dental Medicine,
Harvard University and
Massachusetts Citizens' Committee
for Dental Health,
Boston, Massachusetts
Figures 2a, 2b

Richard H. Lyons, M.D.
State University of New York
Upstate Medical Center
Syracuse, New York
Figure 33

F. J. Margolis, M.D. *et al.*
Wayne State University,
College of Medicine
Kalamazoo, Michigan
Charts 2, 3, 4, 5

Karl E. Mason, Ph.D.
Bethesda, Maryland
Figures 46a, 46b

Rustin McIntosh, M.D.
Tyringham, Massachusetts
Figure 41

D. S. McLaren, M.D.
American University
of Beirut, Lebanon
and Bull. of World Health Org.
34:357, 1966
Figures 8, 10

Metropolitan Life Insurance Company
New York, New York
Appendix D

C. V. Moore, M.D.
St. Louis, Missouri
Figures 39a, 39b

National Health Education Committee, Inc.
New York, New York and
Department of Health,
Education and Welfare,
National Center for Health Statistics
Washington, D.C.
Chart 1b

Hildery A. Nelson, M.D.
Jamestown, New York
Figures 15, 16a, 16b

Rosa Lee Nemir, M.D.
New York University,
School of Medicine
New York, New York
Figure 43

Anthony J. Radford
Papua Medical College
Kainantuehd,
Territory of Papua
and New Guinea
Figure 4a

Blair C. Rich, D.D.S., F.I.C.D.
Rexburg, Idaho
Figure 23
Charts 6, 7

Carl C. Seltzer, Ph.D.
Department of Nutrition,
Harvard, University
Boston, Massachusetts
Appendix D

Karl Singer, M.D.
Chicago, Illinois
Figures 37a, 37b

Charley Smith, M.D.
University of Colorado
Medical Center
Denver, Colorado
Figure 40

Tom Spies, M.D. and
The Upjohn Company
Figures 25a, 25b, 25c, 27a, 27b, 32a, 32b

John C. Stalker, Director
Office of School Lunch Programs
and Nutrition Education
Department of Education,
Commonwealth of Massachusetts
Boston, Massachusetts
Figure 4d

Fredrick J. Stare, M.D.
School of Public Health,
Department of Nutrition
Harvard University
Boston, Massachusetts
Figures 4b, 5, 9

The Upjohn Company
Kalamazoo, Michigan
Figures 7, 12a, 12b, 13a, 13b,
17a, 17b, 17c, 25a, 25b, 25c,
26a, 26b, 26c, 27a, 27b, 30,
32a, 32b, 36a, 36b, 48a, 48b, 48c